YOUNGER
NEXT WEEK

Your Ultimate Rx to Reverse
the Clock, Boost Energy and Look
and Feel Younger in 7 Days

ELISA ZIED
MS, RD, CDN

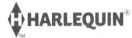

YOUNGER NEXT WEEK

ISBN-13: 978-0-373-89283-9

The health advice presented in this book is intended only as an informative resource guide to help you make informed decisions; it is not meant to replace the advice of a physician or to serve as a guide to self-treatment. Always seek competent medical help for any health condition or if there is any question about the appropriateness of a procedure or health recommendation.

Library of Congress Cataloging-in-Publication Data
Zied, Elisa.
    Younger next week : your ultimate Rx to reverse the clock, boost energy and look and feel younger in 7 days / Elisa Zied, MS, RD, CDN.
        pages cm
        Includes bibliographical references and index.
    ISBN 978-0-373-89283-9 (alk. paper)
    1. Rejuvenation. 2. Longevity. 3. Aging—Prevention. I. Title.
    RA776.75.Z54 2014
    613.2—dc23
    2013023678

www.Harlequin.com

Printed in U.S.A.

To my parents, Barbara (BB) and Ron (the king of my castle), for their unwavering love and support. And to the three greatest loves of my life, my husband, Brian, and our sons, Spencer and Eli, for allowing me to pursue my passions.

CONTENTS

INTRODUCTION

With our revved-up lifestyles, suddenly precarious career paths, piled-up household duties and the constant pings from our mobile devices, it's no surprise that feeling "stressed out" has become the new normal for too many women in this relatively new century. According to the 2012 *Stress in America* survey by the American Psychological Association, women are more likely than men to say their already high stress levels continue to rise. The survey found that 34 to 45 percent of women in the United States reported that stress makes them feel fatigued, nervous, anxious and overwhelmed. Their high stress levels result in a lack of interest in everyday activities and sap their motivation and energy. Women reported that stress makes them cry, gives them headaches and leaves them sleepless at night, staring at the ceiling. Moreover, 46 percent said they cope with stress by overeating or eating unhealthy foods, and 31 percent said they skip meals to manage stress, which can actually exacerbate stress and affect how women look and feel from day to day.

These results are supported by the nearly one hundred forty-something and older women who responded to my Vitality Survey *(you'll see their stories featured throughout the book, though I've changed their names to keep their identities private)*. More than 50 percent said that when life gets overwhelming, they turn to comfort foods, caffeinated energy boosters, alcohol and other vitality robbers. Some women say they overindulge in high-fat, high-sugar, high-calorie comfort foods (think chocolate, muffins, chips, and good ole mac and cheese). Some guzzle lots of high-calorie coffee drinks (a 460-calorie Java Chip Frappuccino, anyone?), sodas (364 calories in a Big Gulp from 7-Eleven) or energy drinks (three 110-calorie Red Bulls equal a major problem) for a quick pick-me-up.

Other women drink alcohol (three Long Island Iced Teas add up to nearly 900 calories) to calm down. Some women skip meals, and when they finally do eat, they grab cookies, ice cream, candy or even their kids' Goldfish crackers, most often swallowed on the run. While these habits may give us a temporary energy boost or a momentary burst of mental clarity, ultimately they cause us to crash and give rise to fatigue and brain fog. They also may contribute to a bulging waistline, drooping skin and unpredictable mood swings. These methods of coping ultimately increase our body's stress response, leaving us more likely to catch that cold that's going around, and elevate our risk for serious disease.

Do these women sound like you, even a little bit? I wrote *Younger Next Week*—which provides a road map to help you look and feel your best, no matter how challenging, complicated or stressful—to help you feel empowered each and every day, no matter how many curveballs life throws at you. And, true confession, I also wrote it to help myself, a forty-four-year-old "multitasker" with a professional career, a husband and two children. I need *Younger Next Week* as much as you do.

Younger Next Week puts the brakes on vitality sappers and helps you recapture your youthful, energetic, positive spirit. I poured through hundreds of scientific studies (so that you don't have to) about diet, fitness and health to pinpoint what really works. I drew from my experience as a practicing dietitian for nearly twenty years, during which time I've helped hundreds of women, and from my real-life experience as a working mother, a freelance writer, an author and a public speaker, to create the *Younger Next Week* lifestyle plan.

In Part II of this book, the Vitality Program, I share my groundbreaking Vitality Diet, which incorporates Vital Foods in appropriate portions to help you feel physically and mentally energized as you achieve, and maintain, a healthier body weight. When you follow the Vitality Diet, you can rest assured there's a sound scientific foundation for all the recommendations. Based on current science-based dietary guidelines and emerging research, the Vitality Diet is not meant to be a rigid prescription for how to eat, but rather a flexible, realistic plan that you can follow and tweak to meet your personal food preferences and lifestyle. The Vitality Diet includes many of the most common, widely available foods—some that may surprise you—to help make it realistic to follow and easy to maintain. After all, you should not have to buy pricey "fad" foods to eat a vitality-boosting diet.

In Part III of this book, Vitality for Life, I help you put the research and the diet into action with my 7-Day Vitality Plan (outlined in Chapter 12)—yes, you *will* look and feel younger in just one week!—with my delicious kitchen-tested Vital Recipes (see Chapter 13), many of which take fifteen minutes or less to prepare. Along with diet guidance, the 7-Day Vitality Plan features exercise and lifestyle advice designed to decrease stress and increase vitality. (Don't worry. No gym is required.) In Chapter 14, you'll find even more

Vitality Menu Ideas to help you feel satisfied. You'll also find Stressipes (rhymes with *recipes*)—food, fitness and lifestyle remedies—sprinkled throughout the book to help you better manage or cope with stress, the greatest vitality buster, and turn intentions to eat and live better into tangible actions.

On Twitter and Facebook, I encourage women to "move it or lose it" (#moveitorloseit), meaning move more in their regular daily life—not just when they're at the gym or in a fitness class. Staying active is essential for healthy muscles and bones, and it helps dampen your mental and physical response to everyday stressors, which can contribute to those less than healthy coping behaviors. My exercise philosophy is not about staying active to "lose weight"; it's about staying active so you don't "lose" your mind and your sanity. Getting enough sleep is also crucial to a more vital you, and *Younger Next Week* shows you how to eat (and drink) and live in a way that enhances—rather than sabotages—your ability to sleep well.

Whether you are approaching forty years old or are closer to fifty years old (or are north of that), my goal in sharing *Younger Next Week* is to help you feel your best, no matter your age. So, with thanks and much love, I present you with *Younger Next Week*. I sincerely hope that after reading my book and applying its food, fitness, and lifestyle principles to your life each and every day, you move—without trepidation or fear, but with excitement—toward, dare I say, embracing and celebrating your age on each birthday you're blessed to enjoy.

At forty-four years old, I feel better than ever. By using the tools in *Younger Next Week,* so can you. You are truly in the driver's seat when it comes to the way you view the world and live your life—even when things seem to be out of control. It's up to you to nourish, care for and preserve your body, your soul and your mind the best way you can, and to see yourself as someone who is truly worth more than her weight—or age—in gold.

~**Elisa**

PART ONE

CHECK YOUR VITAL SIGNS

HAVE YOU LOST YOUR VITALITY?

Happy forty-fourth birthday! Yeah, right. When my friend Claire recently rang in this milestone, she told me she felt like it could have been her fifty-fourth birthday, and to be honest, poor Claire was looking a little worn down. It's no surprise why. She constantly runs after three rambunctious and spirited kids under the age of ten, one of whom has ADHD and always gets into trouble at school. Some days Claire says she feels like a designated taxi driver, shuttling all her kids to and from school, soccer practices and playdates, and her special needs son to and from medical appointments. Her husband, who finally found a new job after being out of work for two years, brings home less than half his former salary. Because he's also trying to get a new side business off the ground, he isn't around to help much with the kids. Claire has managed to hang on to her job as a nurse but puts in longer hours to help make ends meet. On top of all that, her mother-in-law, who suffers from early-stage dementia, has lived with them for the past three years. No wonder Claire feels older than her age and isn't looking her best! To cope, Claire downs a six-pack of diet soda just to make it through each day and munches through an entire family-size bag of corn chips in the evenings. What was her birthday wish? Claire said she wanted a face-lift—for her life!

Claire isn't alone. Just look at Marsha. For years, this forty-five-year-old married mother of two has been in a rut that she can't seem to climb out of. About forty pounds overweight, she works all day as a store clerk and comes home to a nightly routine of homework, baths and "Mama this" and "Mama that," which really take a toll on her nerves. She often asks herself, *Don't my kids have a Daddy?* because her husband helps out with the kids and the household chores only when she asks him. Feeling like she has to nag him makes her resentful and rarely puts her in the mood for intimacy, which adds yet another layer of stress. Although Marsha tries to sneak in thirty minutes of exercise in between work and picking her kids up from their grandmother's house after school, her son now wants to be picked up earlier—so there goes her exercise! She blames herself for her excess weight, but with so many worries and tasks weighing her down and so little time for herself, she drowns her sorrows in sweets, diet soda and beer to unwind over the weekends. Who can blame her?

Susan, a successful architect who owns her own design firm, is in a vitality rut. After weathering a painful divorce and a couple of scary lean years getting her business off the ground, Susan, who just turned forty, thought that turning a decade older would mark the beginning of a fresh chapter in her life. Instead, her packed days spent managing her office, meeting with clients and traveling leave her with little time to exercise or eat. She usually skips breakfast and noshes on nuts, dried fruit, cookies and power bars throughout the day, when she remembers to. At night, if she's not out for dinner with clients (or, on occasion, friends), she collapses at home with take-out food and a glass or two of wine. But she always has trouble falling asleep: her mind races with business ideas and items to add to her next day's "to do" list. Recently, on an outing with her "best buddy," her ten-year-old nephew, she was startled when he asked, "Aunt Susan, are you mad or just tired?" She said she "felt neither," but she later raced to the bathroom mirror and, sure enough, saw a "too-skinny lady" with dark circles under her eyes and what appeared to be permanent frown lines etched into her forehead. *Is it time to visit Dr. Botox?* she joked to herself—but it wasn't really funny.

And then there's me. Always the optimist, I entered my forties with a bang, but the bubble burst quickly. A nagging, painful wrist injury slowed me down, so I couldn't exercise, couldn't cook and couldn't even hold my children's hands. But my wrist was only one of my many stressors. My amazing, hardworking husband, Brian, had recently left his stable job—in the midst of an economic crisis, mind you—to launch his own business in a highly competitive, dog-eat-dog industry. Sure, I was excited for him, but a little terrified, too. Okay, a lot terrified. Then, when I made a routine visit to the dermatologist, my doctor discovered a suspicious mole on my lower back, which was biopsied and ultimately removed. Could it be skin cancer? And then, just before my wrist surgery, my gynecologist found something she didn't like on my mammogram, and I scheduled a biopsy for two weeks after my wrist surgery. OMG, did I have breast cancer? Thankfully, Brian's business is now doing well (knock on wood), the mole was only precancerous and the breast biopsy turned out to be nothing to worry about. But even though things were "okay" on the surface, I saw several close friends go through personal crises—health scares, job losses, marriage troubles, deaths of family members and money struggles—and these crises took an emotional toll on them and me, and I became a frazzled mess.

I started feeling old and debilitated. I had always been active, energetic and vibrant, and for the first time, I felt sidelined. Normally an upbeat, glass-half-full type of gal, I was feeling extremely blue. I was also increasingly irritable and didn't want to socialize much, and I sometimes would burst into tears for absolutely, positively "no reason." Plus, I looked perpetually tired. Was I suffering from "post-traumatic forty disorder"? Like so many women in their forties, fifties and beyond, I had lost my vitality.

HAVE YOU LOST YOUR VITALITY?

How about you? Is the daily grind taking its toll? Do you have too much on your plate, too many commitments and too much responsibility? Are you getting bombarded from every angle by several emergencies at once—an unexpected last-minute deadline, a sick child and a fender bender all in the same day? Do you look and feel run-down, overworked, overstressed, and... gulp!... old? If so, you're riding on a speeding train to aging. Emerging evidence based on Nobel Prize–winning research suggests that chronic stress—the kind we women face on a daily basis—causes premature aging at the cellular level, effectively rendering your body, including your skin, face and hair, up to ten years older than you really are (see Stress Ages You!). It all adds up to wrinkles, sagging skin and an expanding waistline—the telltale signs that your vitality has gone MIA.

Stress Ages You!

In 2004 it was discovered that chronic stress promotes cellular aging. In a study published in *Proceedings of the National Academy of Sciences,* researchers compared thirty-nine premenopausal women between the ages of twenty and fifty who cared for chronically ill children for one to twelve years and nineteen premenopausal women who cared for healthy children. Not surprisingly, those who cared for the sick children reported higher levels of perceived stress. The researchers found that women who had the highest levels of perceived stress had telomeres–the protective caps found on DNA, the body's basic genetic material–that, on average, were shorter by the equivalent of at least one decade of aging compared to low-stress women. The high-stress women also had higher levels of oxidative stress, another marker of aging.

There's no doubt that many of us women who are forty-something or beyond are over-worked, overstretched and overwhelmed. Plus, as many as one in five of us possess the "type D personality" and thus have a propensity to feel anxious, irritable, overly critical or negative or to be socially withdrawn (the D stands for "distressed"), which makes us even more vulnerable to the stresses of daily life. Even those of us who don't fit that profile and seem "so together" may, in fact, possess some of the type D personality traits at least some of the time. That, too, makes us more susceptible to a worn appearance, chronic fatigue, a bad attitude and other negative symptoms that can come from life in the pressure cooker.

There's no denying it—many of us feel like we have lost our vitality, and we look and feel older than we actually are. Many women cope by racing to the nearest cosmetics counter for the latest wrinkle cream, enduring Botox injections and chemical peels, or visiting a plastic surgeon for a more extreme makeover. But there's a much easier, more powerful, less costly, absolutely painless and much more satisfying way to reclaim your vitality.

You are much better off trading in the plastic surgeon's scalpel for a knife and fork. Seriously, one of the most important things you can do to reclaim your vitality and live your absolute best, most fulfilled life is to make tweaks in your food and nutrient intake. Drawing on the most up-to-date science and my vast experience as a registered dietitian for almost two decades, I will show you that beyond a doubt, eating certain foods can be a one-way ticket to vitality. Incorporate these foods into your diet as part of your 7-Day Vitality Plan (see Chapter 12) and you will look and feel younger. With this no-hassle comprehensive plan and the Stressipes sprinkled throughout the book, you can flip the switch on aging and be well on your way toward enjoying boundless energy, supercharged health, a sexier body, a better mood and better sex—in just seven days.

THE VITALITY DIET

In *Younger Next Week,* I offer a simple guide to eating that will help you look and feel more vibrant, more energized and more alive. As a registered and certified dietitian and nutritionist, I know that our diets play a huge role in our ability to achieve, regain, and maintain physical and mental vigor and physical and emotional endurance—in other words, our *vitality*. Based on almost two decades of experience and the most current scientific research, I have targeted the foods, drinks and nutrients that will help you achieve what I call the "7 Pillars of Vitality." These are:

- **A radiant appearance.** Slow down the aging clock and say hello to a more youthful you with smoother skin, a brighter complexion, shinier hair, stronger nails and more.

- **Boundless energy—physical, mental and sexual.** Leap out of bed in the morning, power through your day and still feel revved up for date night (or just some downtime) with your significant other.

- **Brighter moods and emotional fortitude.** Say buh-bye to the blahs, the blues, and mood swings and gain emotional strength to effectively handle hassles without "losing it."

- **Effortless weight management.** Get your comfort eating and snacking under control to slim down or prevent weight gain, and learn about the right foods to eat when stressed. At the same time, learn how to avoid unhealthy weight loss that makes your face pay the price with premature sagging and wrinkling.

- **Better memory and cognition.** Feel more mentally sharp and enjoy better brain function to stay on your game at work and at home. No more misplacing your keys!

- **A sense of calm and relaxation.** Chill when you need to, relax and be ready to fall asleep faster, stay asleep longer, and wake up looking and feeling refreshed.

- **Supercharged health and well-being.** Strengthen your immunity and reduce inflammation to slow aging and live longer and better by reducing the risks of chronic disease and susceptibility to colds, flu and infection.

When you possess the 7 Pillars of Vitality, you can't help but feel vibrant, invigorated and rejuvenated. The Vital Foods I discuss in this book—including delicious options like popcorn, salmon, edamame and even, believe it or not, jelly beans!—have amazing stress-busting, mood-boosting, energy-pumping, age-defying properties that can help you rediscover your vitality.

The beauty of the Vitality Diet is that it's flexible, so busy women can easily follow it. For those of you who want more energy and more vibrancy starting today, I've created a jump-start 7-Day Vitality Diet that incorporates nutritious, delicious foods, which are outlined in the Vital Foods List (see Chapter 12), and includes mouthwatering Vital Recipes, which you'll find in Chapter 13. For even more flexibility and variety, you'll find more meal and snack options, which you can mix and match, in Chapter 14.

But living an all-around life of vitality involves more than watching just what and how much you eat. How you live is equally important. The 7-Day Vitality Plan includes daily and weekly goals to help you move it, lift it, laugh it off, connect, reflect and sleep it off. All these key components work synergistically to help you learn to love and celebrate the skin you're in and unleash a more vibrant you.

CHECK YOUR VITAL(ITY) SIGNS QUIZ

Because it's critical to have a map, or a GPS, to guide you on a new road trip, it's crucial to know exactly where you're starting from now, and where you're headed, before embarking on any adventure. To help you assess where you are now in terms of your food, fitness, and lifestyle behaviors and to check your vitality, I've come up with a ten-minute quiz.

1   **How many portions of whole grains do you eat on a typical day? (1 portion = 1 cup whole-grain cereal, 3 cups air-popped popcorn, 5 Triscuits, ½ cup cooked whole-wheat pasta, ½ cup cooked brown or wild rice)**
    (A) 0   (C) 2
    (B) 1   (D) 3 or more

2   **How much fruit (not including juice) do you eat on a typical day? (½ cup = half a medium banana, ½ cup berries, 16 grapes, 1 small orange, half a grapefruit)**
    (A) 0   (C) 1 cup
    (B) ½ cup   (D) 1½ cups or more

3   **How many cups of colorful non-starchy vegetables (not including corn, potatoes, green lima beans and green peas) do you eat daily?**
    (A) 0   (C) 1½-2 cups
    (B) ½-1 cup   (D) >2 cups

4   **How many nuts/seeds do you eat on a typical day? (½ ounce = 12 almonds, 14 peanuts [technically legumes], 7 walnut halves, 24 pistachios, about 2 tablespoons seeds)**
    (A) 0   (C) 1 ounce
    (B) ½ ounce   (D) at least 1½ ounces

5   **How much fish do you eat during a typical week? (3 ounces = the size of a checkbook or a deck of cards)**
    (A) 0   (C) 7-9 ounces
    (B) 3-6 ounces   (D) 10-12 ounces

6   **How many cups of beans/peas do you eat each week?**
    (A) 0   (C) 1 cup
    (B) ½ cup   (D) at least 1½ cups

7 **How many cups of nonfat or low-fat milk/yogurt or calcium-fortified soy beverages do you consume daily?**
   (A) 0
   (B) 1 cup
   (C) 2 cups
   (D) 3 cups

8 **How many alcoholic drinks do you have weekly? (1 drink = 5 ounces wine, 12 ounces beer, 1½ ounces distilled spirits, such as gin or vodka)**
   (A) 0
   (B) 1-4
   (C) 5-7
   (D) more than 7

9 **How many calories from sugary beverages or snacks or from snack chips would you estimate you consume daily? (50 calories = 4 ounces soda, 1 chocolate chip or Oreo cookie, 15 plain M&M'S, 4 peanut M&M'S, 2 Hershey's Kisses, 20 Goldfish, 4 Doritos, 1 tablespoon table sugar)**
   (A) 50 calories
   (B) 51-100 calories
   (C) 101-150 calories
   (D) more than 150 calories

10 **Do you overeat (eat past the point of fullness, to where you're uncomfortable)? If so, how often?**
   (A) never
   (B) 1-3 times a week
   (C) 4-6 times a week
   (D) at least once a day

11 **How many 8-ounce cups of fluid do you drink daily (not counting alcoholic beverages)?**
   (A) 0-2
   (B) 3-4
   (C) 5-6
   (D) at least 7-8

12 **How many times a week do you do at least 30 minutes of aerobic exercise (e.g., walking, jogging or running; biking; swimming; dancing; or playing sports like tennis or basketball)?**
   (A) 0
   (B) 1-2
   (C) 3-4
   (D) 5-6

13 **How many days per week do you do muscle-strengthening exercise for at least 20 minutes?**
   (A) 0
   (B) 1
   (C) 2
   (D) 3 or more

14 **How many hours do you sleep on a typical night?**
- Ⓐ less than 6
- Ⓒ 7-9
- Ⓑ 6-7
- Ⓓ more than 9

15 **How often do you feel stressed?**
- Ⓐ never
- Ⓒ 1-6 times a week
- Ⓑ once a day
- Ⓓ several times a day

16 **Which of the following best describe what you typically do when you feel stressed? (Circle all that apply.)**
- Ⓐ I listen to music
- Ⓒ I eat/drink
- Ⓑ I call a friend
- Ⓓ I exercise

17 **How often do you laugh?**
- Ⓐ never
- Ⓒ 4-6 times a week
- Ⓑ 1-3 times a week
- Ⓓ daily

18 **How often do you connect with others, not counting by email or social media (e.g., have lunch or do an activity with a friend, volunteer, write a letter)?**
- Ⓐ never
- Ⓒ 4-6 times a week
- Ⓑ 1-3 times a week
- Ⓓ daily

19 **How often do you take even just 15 minutes to do nothing except reflect and relax (e.g., meditate, write in a journal, sit quietly)?**
- Ⓐ never
- Ⓒ 4-6 times a week
- Ⓑ 1-3 times a week
- Ⓓ daily

20 **How often do you look in the mirror and feel good about the way you look?**
- Ⓐ never
- Ⓒ 4-6 times a week
- Ⓑ 1-3 times a week
- Ⓓ daily

21 **Which of the following best describes how old you feel?**
- Ⓐ I feel older than I am
- Ⓒ It varies
- Ⓑ I feel my age
- Ⓓ I feel younger than I am

Give yourself the following number of points for each of your responses:

	A	B	C	D	Your score:
1	Ⓐ = 0	Ⓑ = 1	Ⓒ = 2	Ⓓ = 3	______
2	Ⓐ = 0	Ⓑ = 1	Ⓒ = 2	Ⓓ = 3	______
3	Ⓐ = 0	Ⓑ = 1	Ⓒ = 2	Ⓓ = 3	______
4	Ⓐ = 0	Ⓑ = 1	Ⓒ = 2	Ⓓ = 3	______
5	Ⓐ = 0	Ⓑ = 1	Ⓒ = 2	Ⓓ = 3	______
6	Ⓐ = 0	Ⓑ = 1	Ⓒ = 2	Ⓓ = 3	______
7	Ⓐ = 0	Ⓑ = 1	Ⓒ = 2	Ⓓ = 3	______
8	Ⓐ = 3	Ⓑ = 2	Ⓒ = 1	Ⓓ = 0	______
9	Ⓐ = 3	Ⓑ = 2	Ⓒ = 1	Ⓓ = 0	______
10	Ⓐ = 3	Ⓑ = 2	Ⓒ = 1	Ⓓ = 0	______
11	Ⓐ = 0	Ⓑ = 1	Ⓒ = 2	Ⓓ = 3	______
12	Ⓐ = 0	Ⓑ = 1	Ⓒ = 2	Ⓓ = 3	______
13	Ⓐ = 0	Ⓑ = 1	Ⓒ = 2	Ⓓ = 3	______
14	Ⓐ = 0	Ⓑ = 2	Ⓒ = 3	Ⓓ = 2	______
15	Ⓐ = 3	Ⓑ = 2	Ⓒ = 1	Ⓓ = 0	______
16	Ⓐ = 1	Ⓑ = 1	Ⓒ = 0	Ⓓ = 1	______
17	Ⓐ = 0	Ⓑ = 1	Ⓒ = 2	Ⓓ = 3	______
18	Ⓐ = 0	Ⓑ = 1	Ⓒ = 2	Ⓓ = 3	______
19	Ⓐ = 0	Ⓑ = 1	Ⓒ = 2	Ⓓ = 3	______
20	Ⓐ = 0	Ⓑ = 1	Ⓒ = 2	Ⓓ = 3	______
21	Ⓐ = 0	Ⓑ = 1	Ⓒ = 2	Ⓓ = 3	______
				Total score:	______

What your score means:

If your score is 0–20: Time for a vitality makeover! Your vital(ity) signs are a little weak, but don't despair! The principles outlined in *Younger Next Week* will help you eat more Vital Foods (including whole grains, vegetables, fruits, fish and low-fat dairy), do more Vital Moves (how about some Zumba, hula hooping or jumping rope?) and get the Vital Relaxation you need to help you achieve maximal vibrance.

If your score is 21–49: Your vital(ity) signs aren't weak, but they're not screaming "Vitality now," either. Maybe you just need a few tweaks in your diet (like adding an extra daily serving of whole grains, consuming four extra ounces of fish weekly or drinking two more cups of water daily). Perhaps you need to increase your physical activity, or maybe you need some tools to help you curb your alcohol intake or get a better handle on whatever (or whoever) adds stress to your life.

If your score is 50–60: Your vital(ity) signs are strong, but there's always room for improvement, right? Even if you're doing well in terms of your food, fitness and life-style behaviors (and kudos to you if you are), you can still take steps over the next ten years to lay the foundation for looking and feeling your best, especially as your body continues to change and the M word—menopause—eventually strikes. The principles of the Vitality Diet and the 7-Day Vitality Plan provide the effective ammunition you'll need to fight the physical and emotional challenges that come your way.

COPING HABITS THAT SABOTAGE YOUR VITALITY

When the kids are screaming, a deadline is looming, your bank account is dwindling way too fast, you're fighting a nasty cold and you can barely drag yourself out of bed, what do you do? Let me guess. You reach for chocolate, a bag of chips or a box of cookies. Maybe you race to the nearest Starbucks for a grande Mocha Frappuccino. Maybe you have an extra glass of merlot—okay, make that an extra two...or three glasses—with dinner. Maybe you're so busy, you can't find the time to eat anything and you end up skipping meals completely. If you're like most women, you probably cope with daily or chronic stressors more often than you'd like to with some kind of food or drink that ends up sapping your vitality even more.

HOW WE COPE

Based on the latest scientific evidence, as well as the responses from the nearly one hundred women who took my Vitality Survey, I have identified several common coping habits involving food and eating that strip us of our vitality and age us in so many ways.

OVEREATING

There's evidence that overeating not only contributes to obesity but may also, according to Elizabeth Blackburn, PhD, a Nobel Prize—winning pioneer in telomere research, lead to accelerated aging through the shortening of telomeres, the protective caps at the end of your chromosomes (which are similar to the plastic ends of a shoelace). Overeating can also contribute to elevated cortisol and insulin levels and the suppression of certain hormones, like growth hormone, which may be linked to more rapid aging or a shortened lifespan. It also can contribute to higher blood sugar levels and can promote the premature aging of your face.

A study published in the journal *AGE* in 2013 investigated the link between glucose metabolism and perceived age, as measured by facial photographs of middle-aged subjects. For the first time, researchers found a link between blood sugar levels and facial aging: adults with high blood sugar levels tended to look older compared to those with low blood sugar levels. Although the exact mechanisms by which glucose levels accelerate aging are unclear, the formation of advanced glycation end products (AGEs) is believed to play a role. These substances may prevent the efficient repair of collagen (which plays a role in premature skin aging), may reduce skin elasticity, and may negatively affect collagenous body tissues, such as the heart and kidneys, thereby promoting disease. High glucose levels may also give rise to higher levels of reactive oxygen species, including free radicals (see Chapter 8), which can cause premature cell aging.

Overeating that leads to excess body fat also contributes to inflammation, which, in turn, can dampen the body's immune function and increase the risk of developing chronic diseases, such as heart disease, cancer and diabetes.

CAVING IN TO CRAVINGS

It's no surprise that giving in to cravings—especially when that means eating big portions of high-fat, sugary or salty foods—can weigh you down by adding extra pounds to your body. Emerging evidence suggests this habit may even alter brain chemicals and contribute to withdrawal symptoms when you stop.

In a 2012 study published in the *International Journal of Obesity,* researchers found brain changes in mice who ate a high-fat, high-sugar diet. When the mice stopped consuming that diet, they experienced symptoms of anxiety and depression. Another trigger for the buildup of AGEs, one that wreaks havoc, is drowning your sorrows in comfort foods, such as French fries, or overdoing sugary desserts. Here, AGEs create oxidative stress and inflammation that alter the structure and function of body proteins and increase the risk of diabetes and cardiovascular disease. Studies also suggest that the accumulation of AGEs in skin elastin and collagen interferes with normal skin function and may promote skin aging.

DIETING

When stress hits, rather than indulging themselves, some women may become too rigid and restrictive in their efforts to control their diet and their environment. They cut too many foods, food groups and/or calories from their diet and become overly concerned about everything that passes their lips. Going too far can lead to rapid weight loss, but losing too much weight—especially body fat—too fast not only can de-energize you but can also shift facial aging into high gear. In fact, some research shows that the loss of fat may contribute more to facial aging, sagging and wrinkling than the pull of gravity!

In a 2009 study published in *Plastic and Reconstructive Surgery,* 186 pairs of identical twins completed questionnaires and were photographed. A panel reviewed the images and noted differences in the twins' perceived ages and their facial features. The perceived age differences were then correlated with multiple factors. Among the pairs of twins, the heavier twin looked significantly older than the thinner twin...if they were under the age of forty. But if they were older than forty, the results were reversed, and the thinner twin looked significantly older.

Dieting can also cause feelings of stress and anxiety (not to mention hunger), can wreak havoc on blood sugar levels and can sap much-needed energy. Eating too little can lead to nutritional deficiencies, which have their own sets of health consequences. To make things worse, studies suggest that being overly restrictive when it comes to eating—or merely having the intention to restrict intake—may not only increase psychological stress and promote weight gain, but may also shorten telomeres and accelerate the aging of the immune system.

At one time or another, many women turn to food for comfort or use food as a means to cope during tough times. And while doing that occasionally isn't cause for worry, eating disorder expert Laura Cipullo, RD, CDE, says that using food and eating too often as a way to "gain control" or "numb feelings" may be a red flag for disordered eating or may signal an eating disorder, such as anorexia, bulimia, binge eating disorder or an unspecified eating disorder. "Eating and food should be viewed in a positive way—as equal parts self-care, health and pleasure," Cipullo says. If you fear that your relationship with food is becoming unhealthy, Cipullo suggests educating yourself on the warning signs and risks of disordered eating and eating disorders. And she urges you to be proactive and to seek out a certified eating disorder specialist to help you assess your relationship with food, your body and your life. She notes, "The earlier you receive help, the more likely you are to recover, regain health and learn to eat smart, but intuitively."

NIGHTTIME EATING

There's some proof that those late-night refrigerator raids after a long, stressful day aren't doing you any good. In a study published in *Obesity* in 2011, those who consumed more calories at dinner and after 8:00 p.m. had a higher intake of fast food and full-calorie soda and a lower intake of fruits and vegetables, and they were likely at a higher risk for obesity. Another study published in 2011, this one in the *Journal of Clinical Sleep Medicine*, found that among healthy men and women, higher food intake close to bedtime (within thirty to sixty minutes of hitting the sheets) was associated with negative effects on sleep quality, especially among women. According to Kelly Allison, PhD, an assistant professor in the Department of Psychiatry at the Perelman School of Medicine at the University of Pennsylvania, there's mounting evidence from animal studies that suggests that our bodies do not process food as efficiently when it is eaten at night. Allison says, "Although rodents typically eat at night, when they shift that pattern and eat during the day instead (when they are supposed to be sleeping), they gain more weight and store more fat compared to rodents who eat during their usual time at night." Although more studies are needed to show a similar effect in humans, Allison says studies of the effects of eating at night cite a higher storage of fat, increases in cholesterol and the impaired processing of glucose.

SKIPPING MEALS

When things get overwhelming, some women tend to lose their appetite and skip meals—especially when they run on adrenaline during the day. But often hunger will eventually take over, and they'll make up for those calories (and then some) around dinnertime. But even if their total daily calorie load remains the same, they may be setting themselves up for potentially harmful metabolic changes. In a study that appeared in *Metabolism* in 2007, researchers from the National Institute of Aging found that skipping meals by day and having a large evening meal led to elevated fasting glucose levels and a delayed insulin response, conditions that over time could contribute to diabetes. Skipping meals and waiting too long in between meals can make your blood sugar levels drop and make you feel irritable and sluggish. And when you do finally eat, you may be so hungry that you reach for an ice cream sundae instead of a balanced, vitality-boosting meal.

Vitality Check ✔

Should You Say No to Yo-Yo Dieting?

Some women cope with stress by dieting but then quickly revert to their old unhealthy habits, keeping them on a roller coaster of weight gain and weight loss, which has been shown to slow metabolism and depress the immune system. Years, or even decades, of losing and gaining as little as ten to twenty pounds also robs your skin of the vital elasticity it needs. Here's how: Each time you gain weight, your skin stretches. When you lose weight, your skin has to bounce back to its original shape. Over time, too much stretching damages elastin, a protein in the skin that allows it to snap back into shape. The loss of elastin promotes sagging and drooping. And losing and gaining the same five, ten or twenty pounds repeatedly also takes its toll on your self-esteem and sense of self-worth. So, why not say no to the yo-yo and instead follow the 7-Day Vitality Plan outlined in Chapter 12 to help you not only achieve and maintain a healthier body weight but also have a healthier psyche and feel better about yourself?

DRINKING ALCOHOL

According to the Centers for Disease Control and Prevention (CDC), one in eight American women reports binge drinking (having at least four drinks per sitting), and nearly fourteen million women binge drink three times a month and have an average of six drinks per binge. Besides increasing the risk of breast cancer, heart disease, sexually transmitted diseases and unplanned pregnancy, binge drinking—particularly when it leads to intoxication, hangovers or passing out—has been linked with depressive symptoms. And drinking alcohol in response to stress was shown to actually prolong rather than lessen feelings of tension in a study published in *Alcoholism: Clinical and Experimental Research* in 2011.

Although many factors may contribute to binge drinking, it's likely that stress leads at least some women to go from having a nightly glass of wine to finishing a whole bottle. Besides increasing the risk of chronic diseases, neurological impairments and social problems, drinking too much over time can promote premature aging, which is especially noticeable on your face. Alcohol dehydrates the skin and encourages the formation of more fine lines and wrinkles. But that's not all. It also depletes the body of vitamin A, which is necessary for cell regeneration. And in excessive amounts, alcohol limits the liver's ability to remove toxins, which make you look older. Excess alcohol also compromises immunity. And although studies suggest that drinking has no deleterious effect on body weight and may even be associated with lower body weight (and less weight gain) in women, there are healthier ways to lose weight (or maintain it) *and* gain vitality.

OD'ING ON CAFFEINE

Maybe that once-a-day or once-in-a-while can of caffeinated diet soda has become something you sip on from the first thing in the morning until bedtime, or maybe you rely on several cups of java just to make it through the day. Can you relate? I know I can! But by ingesting that much caffeine, you are shifting the aging process into warp speed. Too much caffeine dehydrates your skin and also interferes with your ability to get restful sleep, which not only drains your energy but also prevents the essential cell regeneration and skin repair that occur primarily at night. Drinking coffee, caffeinated sodas or energy drinks nonstop not only has potential health perils but can also keep you, and your stress, buzzing in high gear.

HOW TO RESTORE, RECLAIM AND REJUVENATE YOUR LIFE

If you frequently OD on cupcakes, skip meals or have one too many cocktails to manage your stress, know you're not alone—especially if you're a woman. We all sink into less than healthful coping habits at least some of the time. But now that you see how some of the less than healthy ways you cope with daily or chronic stress take their toll on your vibrancy, you're likely ready to move toward reclaiming your energy and youthful spirit. Help is on the way! In Part II you'll learn all about the key components of the Vitality Diet and how to eat and drink in a way that keeps you refreshed and energized by day and relaxed by night. You'll also learn about the Vital Moves that help you look and feel younger and how Vital Relaxation can help you reclaim and sustain your vibrancy.You'll also find Stressipes—food, fitness and lifestyle remedies—sprinkled throughout the chapters to help you flip some of your go-to coping habits into ones that help you achieve and preserve the 7 Pillars of Vitality.

PART TWO

THE VITALITY PROGRAM

CHAPTER

3

SETTLE DOWN WITH STARCHY CARBS (AND A SPOONFUL OF SUGAR)

For years starchy carbs—especially "white foods," like pasta, potatoes and white bread—have been under attack. They have been collectively blamed for causing everything from bloat and weight gain to type 2 diabetes and even acne, and experts and consumers alike continue to debate the role, if any, that starchy carbs should have in a healthful diet. Unfortunately, the confusion and lack of consensus among experts has no doubt led many forty-something women to relegate starchy carbs to a nutritional no-man's-land. But while eating these foods or any others beyond your needs and at the expense of healthful foods is never a good idea, especially if it's vibrancy you're looking for, there are many reasons why incorporating starchy carbs, particularly high-fiber whole grains and potatoes, into your Vitality Diet can help you look and feel your very best.

CARBOHYDRATES UNZIPPED

Before we get "up close and personal" with the vital starchy carbs, let's first take a look at how carbohydrates play a key role in the Vitality Diet.

THEY ENERGIZE YOU

Carbohydrates are the ultimate energizers that your brain, your red blood cells, your entire nervous system and your muscles rely on. When you consume carbohydrate-rich foods, such as bread, oatmeal, potatoes, beans, fruit, milk or table sugar, the carbohydrates are broken down into glucose. Although the carbohydrates in whole grains, such as whole-wheat bread or oatmeal, are broken down more slowly (and therefore these foods fill you up more and prevent blood sugar swings) than the carbohydrates found in refined grains, such as white bread or table sugar, the end result is still glucose. And your body—especially your brain—needs glucose to function. Getting it more slowly from whole grains, starchy vegetables, and beans and peas is best, however.

Do 'Em or Ditch 'Em?

Refined Grains

Whole grains trump refined grains when it comes to nutrition, but does eating refined grains do harm? In a 2012 review in *Nutrition Reviews,* researchers examined 135 studies published over a ten-year period, and most found no associations between refined-grain intake and cardiovascular disease, diabetes, weight gain or even death. Although some studies suggest that a very high intake of refined grains might increase the risk of some cancers, the risks were not significant with a moderate intake. Researchers found that consuming up to half of all grains in the form of refined grains (those made without high levels of added fat, sugar or sodium) was not associated with any increased disease risk. Because women currently overdo refined grains, eating about six ounce-equivalents daily (an ounce-equivalent is a slice of white bread or half a cup of cooked pasta), and don't get enough whole grains, eating less than one ounce-equivalent daily, the Vitality Diet calls for women to consume at least four to five starchy carbs daily. Of these, at least three should be whole grains, as advocated by the current Dietary Guidelines for Americans. The rest of the starchy carb alottment can come from refined grains (or even better, potatoes) to meet your daily quota (see Chapter 12).

When your intake of carbohydrate-rich foods is too low and fails to meet minimal needs, your body goes straight to using stored body fat to generate energy. While that doesn't sound like a bad thing, eventually going too low for too long causes your body to break down protein in foods and *you,* including your muscles, to create glucose to feed the brain. This scenario poses a problem, especially because you want to preserve your muscle mass as you get older to keep your body strong and healthy and to keep your metabolic rate supercharged. Also, if you use fat and protein to create energy, it means that those substances aren't able to efficiently execute their many unique functions. Extremely low carbohydrate diets also can cause vitality-sapping side effects, including extreme fatigue, irritability, headaches, dehydration, muscle cramps and poor brain function. Preventing these adverse effects alone make it a no-brainer to include a good dose of carbohydrates from starchy carbs and other sources in any Vitality Diet.

Vitality Check ✔

How Much Carbohydrate Do You Need Daily?

According to the Institute of Medicine's Acceptable Macronutrient Distribution Range (AMDR), which takes into account the total diet and the number of calories people consume based on their weight, height, activity level, body frame and other variables, carbohydrates should represent anywhere from 45 percent to 65 percent of total calories, or about half to two-thirds of your total daily intake. To meet minimal glucose needs for the brain, the National Academy of Science's Recommended Dietary Allowance (RDA) for carbohydrates is 130 grams,* or about 520 calories. To put this in perspective, over the course of a day that's the amount of carbohydrates found in:

1 cup Cheerios with 1 cup nonfat milk · 1 cup nonfat Greek yogurt topped with 2 tablespoons raisins · 1 cup blueberries · 3 cups air-popped popcorn · ½ cup cooked brown rice · 1 cup cooked spinach.

If you are active or are an athlete, you need even more carbohydrates to fuel your hardworking muscles.

*Each gram of carbohydrate provides four calories.

THEY CALM YOU

Carbohydrates are also critical because they provide your body with a steady stream of serotonin. This brain chemical, a type of neurotransmitter, plays a key role in regulating mood, appetite/satiety and sleep. When you eat carbohydrate-rich foods, your blood sugar level rises. This leads to the release of the hormone insulin. Insulin then paves the way for the amino acid tryptophan to pass into the brain. Once in the brain, tryptophan produces serotonin. According to *The Serotonin Power Diet,* by Judith J. Wurtman, PhD, signs of *decreased* serotonin activity in the brain include grumpiness, irritability, impatience, fatigue, an inability to focus, depression and anger. According to Wurtman, "Having a craving for carbohydrate may also indicate that serotonin levels in the brain have fallen."

Vitality Check ✔

Can You Have the Cake You Crave and Eat It, Too?

We all know that cookies, cake and French fries aren't at the top of any Vital Foods List, and for good reason. But does that mean you have to just say no when you crave them? According to David L. Katz, MD, director of the Yale University Prevention Research Center, while you don't have to give up an occasional hunk of chocolate cake or an order of French fries, if you slowly transition to love the foods that love you back (or at least mostly), this can reduce cravings. Here is Katz's three-part strategy to manage cravings.

1. **Arm yourself with all the "right" foods.** The time to start handling a craving is before you get it, by keeping only wholesome foods within reach at all times. Deciding whether to give in to a craving or how to satisfy it *during* the craving is like trying to draft a prenuptial agreement while in *flagrante delicto.*

2. **Rehab your taste buds over time.** Cravings for very sweet or very salty foods occur only if your taste buds *need* very sweet or very salty to register satisfaction. If you dial down your intake of sweet, salty and highly processed foods in general, over time your taste buds will become much more sensitive to flavors; eventually, you'll find you're satisfied by having fewer sweets and less salty foods. You will still get cravings, but they'll be milder, less frequent and easily satisfied with more nutritious foods.

3. **Use the "right" foods to indulge cravings**. Rather than fighting to resist cravings with karate, give in to them—but with judo. Go with the force of the craving, but bend it to your will. For instance, when you crave something sweet, indulge with pure dark chocolate. It will get the job done, and it's also good for you. When you crave something salty, go with a high-quality product, such as organic whole-grain corn chips made from whole-grain corn, canola oil and salt. The less processed the salty food, the less salt it takes for it to taste salty.

THEY AID WEIGHT MANAGEMENT (SURPRISE!)

Carbohydrate intake—especially from fiber-rich sources—also appears to be positively linked with weight management. Consider this:

- A review of several studies published in the *Journal of the American Dietetic Association* in 2007 found that adults who consumed more carbohydrates weighed less than those who consumed fewer carbohydrates. Researchers also noted that those with higher carbohydrate intakes had higher-quality diets than those with lower intakes.

- In a survey of more than forty-four hundred healthy adults, it was found that those who consumed 47 to 64 percent of their total calories in the form of carbohydrates had the lowest risk of being overweight and obese. This 2009 study, published in the *Journal of the American Dietetic Association,* also showed that a lower carbohydrate intake was associated with a greater risk of being overweight and obese.

Diets rich in fiber from starchy carbs and other healthy carbohydrate-rich foods, such as fruits and vegetables, have also been linked with reduced body weight and the prevention of weight gain. According to a 2005 review article in *Nutrition,* population studies provide strong evidence that a higher fiber intake is correlated with lower body weight. Although intervention studies (studies that try to prove cause and effect) have yielded mixed results, the researchers concluded that increasing fiber intake tends to decrease food intake and body weight, in part by promoting satiety.

Fiber is a type of carbohydrate that travels through the body undigested. Fiber has been linked with a reduced risk of coronary heart disease, diabetes and some cancers. It promotes a healthy gastrointestinal system, helps prevent constipation and plays a role in lowering blood cholesterol levels. It also helps regulate blood sugar levels and contributes to a feeling of fullness (and may possibly help with weight management). Emerging research also suggests that fiber may play beneficial roles in immunity and possibly cognition. Unfortunately, women consume on average only about 62 percent of the fiber they need each day—15½ grams—instead of the 25 grams recommended for thirty-one- to fifty-year-olds by the Institute of Medicine. But don't despair. You can easily meet your daily fiber needs—and reap all of fiber's benefits—by consuming fiber-rich whole grains, fruits and vegetables, and beans and peas, as outlined in the Vitality Diet.

START (AND END) YOUR DAY THE WHOLE-GRAIN WAY

Whole grains are vital components of any eating plan because of the vast array of nutrients and beneficial plant chemicals they contain.

What Is a Whole Grain, Anyway?

By definition, a whole grain is composed of three key parts—the bran (the multilayered outer skin, which contains fiber, vitamins, minerals and important plant chemicals), the germ (the embryo of the plant, which contains vitamins, some protein, minerals and fats) and the endosperm (the largest part of the grain, which contains starchy carbohydrates, proteins, vitamins and minerals).

Whole grains, such as oatmeal, brown rice and even popcorn, are rich sources of complex carbohydrates, fiber, and other Vital Nutrients and plant chemicals that play key roles in the body, namely, B vitamins, which help the body create energy from food and support a healthy nervous system; iron, a mineral that carries oxygen throughout the body; and magnesium, a mineral that helps release energy from muscles and build bone.

Whole grains also provide several nutrients that act as antioxidants, which protect cells from harmful chemicals in the environment and in the body, chemicals that both damage cells and contribute to aging and disease. These antioxidants include the mineral selenium, vitamin E, and phytochemicals, such as carotenoids. Other important phytochemicals in whole grains include phenolics (such as flavonoids), γ-oryzanols and beta-glucan.

There's plenty of proof that consuming a diet rich in whole grains boosts vitality by promoting weight management. A study published in the *Journal of Nutrition* in 2012 found strong associations between whole-grain intake and both a lower body mass index and a lower percentage of body fat and abdominal fat in older adults. In a 2010 study that appeared in the *American Journal of Clinical Nutrition,* researchers noted that an increased intake of whole grains was associated with lower visceral fat (which is dangerous fat that accumulates near vital organs) in women. Eating at least one serving of whole grains per day was correlated with a significantly lower body mass index and a lower waist circumference in women compared with eating no whole grains, according to a 2008 study published in the *Journal of the American College of Nutrition.* In a 2003 study published in the *American Journal of Clinical Nutrition,* Harvard University researchers also found that women who consumed more whole grains consistently weighed less than those who had lower whole-grain intakes.

Whole-grain intake has also been linked with a reduced risk of diet-related diseases and conditions, including heart disease, hypertension and type 2 diabetes. In addition, according to Karen Collins, MS, RD, a nutrition advisor for the American Institute for Cancer Research (AICR), whole grains seem to interfere with cancer development at many different stages. She says, "Some may help turn on tumor suppressor genes and turn off genes that lead to cancer development or its ability to spread." Whole grains' cancer-fighting benefits are likely attributed to their many phytochemicals (including fiber), which have antioxidant and other roles.

Although there are many healthful whole grains from which to choose, some are standouts when it comes to their nutrition content, versatility and convenience. In the following pages, you'll learn about the many virtues of a variety of whole grains, including oats, shredded wheat, brown rice, quinoa and popcorn, and how they play an integral role in your Vitality Diet. (Any mention of brand-name items should not be construed as an implied endorsement.)

Vital Stats: Whole Grains*

Whole Grain	Calories	Total Fat (g)	Protein (g)	Carbohydrate (g)	Sodium (mg)	Sugars (g)	Fiber (g)
Barley, cooked (1/2 cup)	97	0	1.8	22	0	0	3
Brown rice, cooked (1/2 cup)	108	1	2.5	22.5	5	0	1.8
Corn, cooked (1/2 cup)	72	1	2.5	15.6	0	3	1.8
Oats, cooked, regular and quick (1/2 cup)	83	1.8	3	14	5	0	2
Popcorn, air-popped (3 cups)	93	1	3.1	18.7	0	0	3.5
Quinoa, cooked (1/3 cup)	74	1	2.7	13.1	0	<1	1.7
Shredded wheat (1/2 cup)	86	0	2.9	20	0	0	3
Triscuits (5)	100	3.8	2.5	16	150	0	2.5
Whole wheat bread (1 slice)	69	1	3.6	11.6	112	2	1.9
Whole wheat pasta, macaroni, cooked (1/2 cup)	87	0	3.8	18	0	<1	2
Wild rice, cooked (1/2 cup)	83	0	3.3	17.5	0	<1	1.5

*Other whole grains include amaranth, buckwheat, bulgur, whole cornmeal, emmer, farro, Kamut, millet, sorghum, spelt, teff, triticale, whole rye, whole or cracked wheat, and wheat berries.
For more information, visit www.wholegrainscouncil.org.

Source: U.S. Department of Agriculture, Agricultural Research Service. 2012. USDA National Nutrient Database for Standard Reference, Release 25. Nutrient Data Laboratory Home Page, www.ars.usda.gov/ba/bhnrc/ndl.

I Spy a Whole Grain

With so many cereal, bread, cracker and pasta options to choose from, finding whole-grain foods is not always easy. To help you out, the Whole Grains Council created a Whole Grain stamp to indicate that a product contains at least eight grams of whole grains (half of a serving*) and a 100 percent Whole Grain stamp to indicate that a product is entirely whole grain. If you don't see a stamp on a package, the Whole Grains Council urges you to look for the following words in the ingredients list, as they indicate that a product is whole grain: whole-grain [name of grain], whole wheat, whole [other grain],

*Sixteen grams of whole grains counts as one serving of whole grains.

stone-ground whole [grain], brown rice, oats, oatmeal (including old-fashioned oatmeal and instant oatmeal) and wheat berries. While the words *wheat* or *wheat flour, semolina, durum wheat, organic flour, stone-ground* and *multigrain* may accurately describe what's in a food package, the product may be missing some parts of the grain and therefore may not be whole grain. And such ingredients as enriched flour, degerminated corn (corn meal or corn flour), bran and wheat germ aren't considered whole grain.

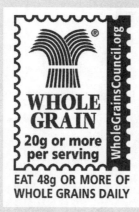 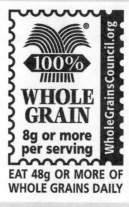

OATS: WHO KNEW?

Consuming oats can play a key role in helping you look and feel younger. They provide carbohydrates that are broken down slowly and gradually released into the bloodstream to keep blood sugar levels steady. This effect is mainly due to the soluble fiber (primarily beta-glucan) they contain. Oats also pack in some protein, which, along with their fiber, can keep you full and satisfied—and possibly prevent overeating, which can contribute to weight gain. Oats contain small doses of healthful monounsaturated and polyunsaturated fats and are low in sodium and sugar and devoid of cholesterol. Consuming cooked oats can even help you and your skin stay hydrated, because of their high water content.

One cup of cooked, unenriched oats is an excellent source of manganese. This mineral helps create energy from protein and carbohydrates, is involved in the synthesis of fatty acids, which is important for a healthy nervous system, and helps make cholesterol to produce sex hormones. It also plays a role in the creation of proteins (including collagen, elastin and cartilage) and helps protect cells in the body against damage from free radicals—highly reactive, unstable molecules that at high levels can harm cells. Manganese also contributes to the formation of gamma-aminobutyric acid (GABA) in the brain, an amino acid that promotes calm and relaxation. Oats are also a good source of Vital Nutrients, such as phosphorus, selenium, magnesium, zinc, thiamine and iron. And oats contain avenanthramides, plant chemicals believed to act as antioxidants and to protect against coronary heart disease, colon cancer and skin irritation.

Oats: A Gift for the Gluten Free?

If you have celiac disease or other conditions that require you follow a diet free of gluten, the protein found in all forms of wheat and in rye, barley and triticale, there's evidence that including oats may boost the nutritional quality of your diet. In a 2010 study published in the *European Journal of Clinical Nutrition*, researchers found that adding oats to the diet helped those with celiac disease increase their intakes of thiamine and magnesium, or magnesium and zinc, when they consumed one hundred grams of oats daily for six months. But given the fact that oats can become cross-contaminated with gluten when manufactured or grown with gluten-containing grains, it's wise to visit the Gluten Free Certification Organization (GFCO) website, www.gluten.net/gfco/default.aspx, to find oats that are certified as gluten free.

Studies have shown that consuming oats can lower several heart disease risk factors, including total cholesterol, LDL (bad) cholesterol and blood pressure. They're believed to exert these benefits because of their beta-glucan content. This soluble fiber has also been shown to aid in the stabilization of blood sugar and to improve insulin sensitivity, thereby reducing type 2 diabetes risk, and also to boost immune function.

I'LL HAVE WHAT SHE'S HAVING! SATISFYING WAYS TO EAT OATS

They don't have to be as plain as your grandmother's oatmeal anymore. Here are some nutritious (and delicious) ways some registered dietitians/nutritionists sweeten or spice up their oats:

- Keri Gans eats Quick Quaker Oats made with nonfat milk and topped with low-fat cottage cheese, cinnamon and chia seeds.

- Elana Tapper Natker makes old-fashioned oats with nonfat milk, frozen berries, chopped almonds and a teaspoon of Splenda Brown Sugar Blend.

- Kate Scarlata loves Bob's Red Mill Steel-Cut Oats topped with berries, chia seeds, pumpkin seeds and a sprinkle of maple sugar.

- Bethany Thayer likes Kroger Quick Oats topped with chopped apple and raisins.

- Delia Willsey enjoys Bob's Red Mill Steel-Cut Oats with almond milk and some peanut butter mixed in.

- Julie Meyer cooks Quaker Old Fashioned Oats with water and a scrambled egg, sometimes adding flaxseed or chia seeds.

Buying and Eating Oats

There are so many different types of oats* to choose from, including steel-cut and rolled varieties. Your healthiest choices are unflavored, low-sodium or no-sodium oats. Quick-cooking or instant oats can save you prep time, but make sure your good-for-you-oats aren't laced with too much sodium and/or sugar. Flavored varieties tend to pack in the most sodium and sugar, so try to sweeten your own unadulterated oats naturally with fresh fruit slices, dried fruit or unsweetened applesauce.

*To learn more about the various types of oats, visit the Whole Grains Council at www.wholegrainscouncil.org/whole-grains-101/types-of-oats.

CEREAL: VITALITY IN A BOX

Whole-grain, high-fiber ready-to-eat cereal is a great vehicle for instant vitality, not only because of the nutrients and beneficial substances it contains, but also because it pairs well with other nutritious, vitality-enhancing foods and beverages, such as milk, fruit and nuts.

Shredded Wheat: The "Super" Cereal

When it comes to cereal, you can't get much better than shredded wheat. It's one of my favorite whole-grain cereals. Not only does shredded wheat provide complex carbohydrates to give you energy, and fiber and protein to fill you up and keep blood sugar levels steady, but it's also low in fat and cholesterol-free. And unlike most ready-to-eat cereals, it's practically devoid of sodium and added sugar. One cup of shredded wheat is also a good source of phosphorus, magnesium and niacin, and it provides small amounts of Vital

continued on page 32

Nutrients, like zinc, thiamine, copper, iron, potassium and folate.

Consider jazzing up your shredded wheat with some fresh berries, sliced banana or dried fruit; chopped walnuts or slivered almonds; and chia seeds or flaxseeds. And if you want to naturally sweeten your cereal, add a sprinkle of sugar.

When it comes to promoting vitality, there's evidence that eating ready-to-eat cereals like shredded wheat boosts nutrient intake. One study published in the *Journal of Aging Research* in 2012 noted that adults aged fifty-five and older who ate ready-to-eat cereal had higher intakes of dietary fiber, whole grains, and several vitamins and minerals than those who did not. A Canadian study that appeared in the *Journal of Nutrition* in 2013 found that eating breakfast—particularly when it included ready-to-eat cereal—was positively associated with better nutrient intake and nutrition status in adults. These findings make sense, since cereal is seldom eaten solo and is often paired with nutrient-rich foods and beverages, such as fresh and dried fruit, nuts and seeds, and low-fat or nonfat milk or yogurt.

Eating ready-to-eat cereal for breakfast—or even after dinner—may also benefit your weight and your waist. Some studies have shown that including cereal with breakfast is linked with a lower body mass index and/or body fat mass. A study published in the *Journal of the American College of Nutrition* in 2012 found that replacing a typical after-dinner snack with ready-to-eat cereal helped overweight habitual evening snackers significantly reduce their nighttime calorie intake. Those who ate cereal at night also consumed substantially fewer calories compared with those who ate their usual nighttime snacks. The researchers concluded that replacing the typical evening snack with ready-to-eat cereal may help overweight people lose weight.

In a study of twenty- to thirty-nine-year-old adults published in *Public Health Nutrition* in 2012, subjects were divided into breakfast skippers, ready-to-eat-cereal eaters and other breakfast eaters based on their twenty-four-hour dietary recalls. Compared with breakfast skippers, cereal eaters were 28 to 42 percent less likely to be overweight/obese and have abdominal obesity, elevated blood pressure, elevated serum total cholesterol, elevated LDL (bad) cholesterol, reduced HDL (good) cholesterol and elevated insulin levels. Those who ate cereal were also 22 percent, 31 percent and 24 percent less likely to be overweight/ obese, have abdominal obesity and have elevated blood pressure, respectively, compared with those who chose other breakfast foods.

The bottom line is that eating cereal—especially whole-grain, high-fiber cereal, like shredded wheat—will likely satisfy you, help you meet your daily quotas for other Vital Foods, such as fruit and dairy, and keep your heart and body weight healthy.

How to Pick Cereal Winners

A walk down any cereal aisle reveals a dizzying display of sugary, flaky, crunchy and crispy options. Since it's challenging to compare cereals in terms of nutritional value due to the fact that serving sizes vary from cereal to cereal, here are some tips to help you cut through the claims on the boxes the next time you shop for cereal:

- **Look for a stamp.** If you can't find a Whole Grain stamp or a 100 percent Whole Grain stamp on the cereal box, look for whole wheat, whole oats or another whole grain listed first in the ingredients list. (See "I Spy a Whole Grain" on page 28.)

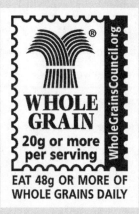 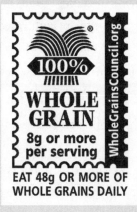

- **Find the fiber.** Aim for at least three grams of fiber for a hundred-calorie portion.
- **Cap the sugar.** A good rule of thumb is to consume cereals with a sugar content of no more than twice the fiber content. So, for every one hundred calories of cereal with three grams of fiber, look for no more than six grams of sugar.
- **Avoid fat traps.** To steer clear of artificial trans fats (which can increase the risk of heart disease, stroke and type 2 diabetes), avoid products that contain such ingredients as shortening or partially hydrogenated vegetable oil. Be aware that some products may list hydrogenated vegetable oil, though technically, it is partially hydrogenated and contains trans fats. Even if the Nutrition

continued on page 34

BROWN RICE: A SUPERSTAR

Rice is one of the most consumed crops in the world. Though rice intake is comparatively low in the United States, there's evidence that making it a regular part of your meals can improve the quality of your diet and help you manage your weight. And the consumption of rice yields other vital health perks. Consider this:

- In a study published in *Nutrition Today* in 2010, researchers looked at national food consumption data and found that, compared with non–rice eaters, those who reported eating at least a quarter cup of cooked white or brown rice daily appeared to eat a more high-quality diet overall. They ate more fruit and legumes (beans and peas, which pair beautifully with rice) and consumed less total fat, saturated fat and added sugars. They also had higher intakes of iron, folate and other B vitamins. An added bonus was that those who regularly ate rice were less likely to be overweight or obese or have risk factors for cardiovascular disease, type 2 diabetes and metabolic syndrome.

- A study that appeared in the *Journal of the American Dietetic Association* in 2009 concluded that rice eaters ate significantly less fat and saturated fat and consumed more iron, potassium, fiber, meat, vegetables and grains than those who didn't eat rice.

- Brown rice may play a role in boosting mood and promoting calm and relaxation. The complex carbohydrates in rice lay the foundation to allow the amino acid tryptophan to pass into the brain, where it produces the "feel-good" brain chemical serotonin. Brown rice is also an excellent source of manganese, a mineral that, among its many key roles, helps activate an enzyme involved in the production of gamma-aminobutyric acid (GABA), an amino acid neurotransmitter that promotes calm and relaxation.

White Rice

Unlike whole-grain brown rice, white rice is a refined grain, stripped of the bran (which packs in fiber, B vitamins and antioxidants) and the germ (which is rich in B vitamins, minerals, protein and healthy fats). White rice also has a higher glycemic index* than brown rice. In a review published in the *British Medical Journal* in 2012, researchers noted that a higher white rice intake was linked with a significantly increased risk of type 2 diabetes. For each daily serving of white rice that subjects ate, type 2 diabetes risk increased by 11 percent. The researchers speculated that the association may be due to how white rice affects the glycemic load** and to the fact that white rice has less insoluble fiber, magnesium, vitamins and beneficial plant chemicals compared with brown rice. Although not all studies agree that white rice is linked with a higher risk of type 2 diabetes (a study published in *Clinical Nutrition* in 2012 even found a lower incidence of type 2 diabetes over six years among those who reported they ate two to three weekly servings of white rice), it's prudent to opt more often for wholesome whole grains over refined ones in your quest for vitality. And when you consume refined grains like white rice, stick to a small portion (half a cup to one cup), and pair it with beans or other lean protein sources to lessen its effects on your blood sugar.

*The glycemic index (GI) is a measure of how fast a particular food raises blood glucose levels compared with the same amount of glucose.

**The glycemic load is a ranking system for the carbohydrate content in foods based on their glycemic index, with portion size taken into account. The glycemic load provides a more accurate indicator of how a particular food will affect blood sugar levels. For instance, some foods that are high on the glycemic index, such as carrots, actually have a low glycemic load once portion size is accounted for. It would take a lot more carrots than potatoes, for instance, to raise your blood sugar the same amount.

NUTRITIONAL BENEFITS OF BROWN RICE

Although all types of rice have virtues—their complex carbohydrates provide energy, and they are practically devoid of fat, cholesterol and sodium—brown rice is a standout. Besides its whole-grain status, it provides fiber (mostly insoluble, the kind that helps treat and prevent constipation) and a little bit of protein, which together help fill you up and stabilize blood sugar levels. A half cup of cooked brown rice is also an excellent source of the mineral manganese and a good source of both magnesium and selenium. In addition, brown rice contains smaller amounts of fourteen other vitamins and minerals.

If that weren't enough, brown rice also boasts potent plant chemicals that may have antioxidant and other protective properties.

Arsenic and Rice: Should I Worry?

In November 2012, *Consumer Reports* reported that brown rice and several other rice products contain arsenic—sometimes in worrisome amounts. Arsenic is naturally found in soil, water, air and food (including grains, fruits and vegetables) and is a by-product of human activity, such as burning coal or using certain pesticides. While it exists in both organic and inorganic forms, inorganic arsenic has been linked with higher rates of cancer and heart disease and cognitive and other developmental disabilities. In a review of two hundred foods, the U.S. Food and Drug Administration (FDA) found high levels of arsenic in rice products; experts at the agency believe that rice takes up more arsenic from the soil and water than other grains. To keep us safe, the FDA recommends consuming a wide variety of grains—and I agree. Mixing up choices from each food group provides you with an array of nutrients and other beneficial substances, and it helps to minimize potentially harmful contaminants in your diet. That strategy can also help reduce boredom—a surefire recipe to help you stick to your Vitality Diet.

QUINOA: THE MOTHER GRAIN

Known as "the mother grain" by the Incas, quinoa (pronounced KEEN-wah) originated in South America, where it has been cultivated and consumed for several thousand years. Despite its nickname, quinoa isn't really a grain, but rather is a grain-like seed that is related to spinach, Swiss chard and beets. This pseudo-grain is often consumed like cereals or rice and is accompanied by lean protein and vegetables. Although it's available in hundreds of varieties and several colors, white/ivory quinoa, with its mild nutty flavor and delicate texture, is the most popular.

QUINOA VITALITY PERKS

Quinoa is a real standout when it comes to plant foods. The United Nations even declared 2013 the International Year of Quinoa because of its incredible nutritional and functional properties. It provides complex carbohydrates for energy and offers a healthy dose of both soluble fiber to help lower cholesterol and insoluble fiber to promote good gastro-intestinal health and prevent constipation. It's also one of the only plant foods besides soybeans that provides high-quality "complete" protein, that is, with all the essential amino acids—the building blocks of protein—which our bodies can't make enough of and derive from our diet. Together, the fiber and protein in quinoa fill us up and help stabilize our blood sugar levels. The little fat that quinoa contains is mostly in the form of heart-healthy polyunsaturated and monounsaturated fats, and it has no cholesterol and is virtually free of added sugar and sodium. One-third cup of cooked quinoa is a good source of manganese and magnesium. It also contains 5 to 10 percent of the Daily Value of phosphorus, folate, copper and iron. Quinoa is also naturally rich in a variety of plant chemicals, many that act as antioxidants to protect cells against free-radical damage.

A 2010 review in the *Journal of the Science of Food and Agriculture* refers to quinoa as an "excellent example of a 'functional food' that may prove to lower disease risk." The article suggests that quinoa's unique combination of minerals, vitamins, fatty acids and antioxidants may protect cell membranes and support brain function, and the authors recommend further study to see if quinoa's antioxidant effects can support memory and reduce stress-induced anxiety. In a 2005 study in the *British Journal of Nutrition,* subjects found quinoa to be more satiating than either wheat or rice. And a study published in the *Journal of Human Nutrition and Dietetics* in 2009 concluded that adding quinoa, a gluten-free grain, to a gluten-free diet improved overall nutrient intake and specifically increased the amounts of protein, iron, calcium and fiber subjects consumed.

7 Quick Quinoa Fixes

"Whether you use white/ivory, red, or black quinoa, the naturally delicious earthy, nutty flavor is the perfect playground for merging other tasty flavors to create unforgettable dishes," says the Bikini Chef herself, Susan Irby, author of *The Complete Idiot's Guide Quinoa Cookbook.* She suggests buying prewashed quinoa or rinsing quinoa in cool water to remove the thin layer of saponins (bitter substances on the outside of the seeds) before cooking. Here are seven ways Irby amps up the flavor of quinoa:

1. **A little bit of spice.** Add cayenne pepper to quinoa for a hot and spicy fix, or go the more savory route with cumin, coriander and curry powder.

2. **Coconut milk.** For a fantastic flavorful variation, cook the quinoa in equal parts coconut milk and water.

continued on page 38

3. **Luscious citrus.** Add fresh lemon, orange, grapefruit or lime zest to quinoa to boost the flavor and color of the quinoa and wake up your taste buds.

4. **Fresh herbs.** Balance out the nuttiness of quinoa by adding minced fresh herbs, such as cilantro, Italian flat-leaf parsley, basil or dill, before serving.

5. **Sweet veggies.** Fold in diced sweet red, yellow or orange bell peppers to impart a vibrant color and a fresh flavor to quinoa.

6. **Black or white pepper.** Add an understated oomph to quinoa with freshly ground black or white pepper.

7. **Sugar au naturel.** Dress quinoa with a simple vinaigrette made with apple cider vinegar, olive oil and a little honey for a naturally sweet and hearty dish. (For 4 cups of cooked quinoa, stir together ½ tablespoon of honey and 2 tablespoons each of vinegar and olive oil. You can also add a small pinch of sea salt and black pepper to the dressing.)

POPCORN

When it comes to snacks, popcorn is a living legend. Popcorn has been enjoyed for thousands of years as both food and fashion: Native American tribes reportedly used it to make necklaces and headdresses. Demand for popcorn soared during the Great Depression because it was cheap and delicious. Popcorn remains popular, especially in movie theaters, where it's usually drenched in oil and coated with salt, making its many virtues fall to the wayside.

POPCORN PERKS

When it comes to nutrition, air-popped popcorn is stellar. This 100 percent whole-grain snack packs in complex carbohydrates to keep you energized, and it contains fiber, particularly insoluble fiber, the kind that aids digestion. It also provides some protein, which, along with fiber, fills you up and stabilizes your blood sugar. Popcorn is naturally low in calories and fat and is virtually free of sodium and sugar.

Think Big *and* Small When You Serve Yourself.

In her book *The Portion Teller Plan,* Lisa Young, PhD, RD, refers to those who eat large portions as "volume eaters." To eat more and stay satisfied while reducing calories consumed, Young urges volume eaters to serve themselves larger portions of lower-calorie, nutrient-packed foods, such as raw, steamed or lightly sautéed non-starchy vegetables and fruit, and smaller amounts of foods that possess a lot of calories in relatively small portions, such as treats, sweets and oils. She also recommends that volume eaters choose fresh fruit over juice, and snacks like air-popped popcorn over pretzels or chips, since these foods pack in fewer calories in relatively large portions.

Besides its other virtues, popcorn supplies more than a dozen healthful vitamins and minerals. Three cups provide a good dose of manganese and smaller amounts of twelve other Vital Nutrients.

Popcorn hulls also boast powerful plant chemicals called polyphenols, even more than are found in fruits and vegetables, according to research by Joe Vinson, PhD, a professor at the University of Scranton. According to a 2012 article in *Critical Reviews in Food Science Nutrition,* depending on their dose and bioavailability, polyphenols can benefit health through their antioxidant, anti-inflammatory and vasodilating (widening of blood vessels) properties. They also may act as probiotics in the gut, promoting "good" bacteria that kill or inhibit the growth of "bad" bacteria and other microorganisms.

Shopping for Popcorn

When you buy popcorn, keep it simple. Opt for plain kernels to pop at home using an air popper. If you're concerned about pesticides or want to avoid genetically modified foodstuffs, buy organic varieties of popcorn. When it comes to bagged popped popcorn, pickings are slim. Although most microwave popcorns are made with unhealthy chemicals (in the bag and in the popcorn) and additives, Quinn Popcorn, a newer brand, uses organic kernels that aren't genetically modified and the popcorn comes in a chemical-free, compostable paper bag. If you don't mind a little extra healthy fat—about the same amount you'd get if you popped the popcorn yourself with a teaspoon or two of oil—two pre-popped,

continued on page 40

bagged options, Skinny Pop Popcorn and Angie's Boom Chicka Pop, each with only three ingredients (popcorn, sunflower oil, and salt or sea salt), fit the bill. And when it comes to the popcorn you find at movie theaters, amusement parks and sports arenas, or the popcorn that arrives in a big gift tin, sample it in small portions as an occasional treat, since it's most likely drenched in oil and salt and/or smothered with sugar—which can turn an otherwise wholesome whole-grain snack into a decadent dessert.

There's some evidence that eating popcorn may be a marker for a more healthful diet. A study that appeared in the *Journal of the American Dietetic Association* in 2008 found that those who reported that they regularly ate a little more than three cups of popped popcorn daily consumed 250 percent more whole grains and 22 percent more fiber than those who did not eat popcorn. Popcorn eaters also tended to eat more grains and less meat, had higher intakes of protein, magnesium and niacin, and had lower intakes of folate. Another study, this one published in *Nutrition Journal* in 2012, found that eating six cups of low-fat popcorn made subjects feel more full over the short term than eating one cup of potato chips. Researchers concluded that popcorn is a prudent snack for those who want to reduce hunger while managing calorie intake and body weight.

Add Pep to Your Popcorn

If the thought of munching on naked air-popped popcorn leaves your taste buds unexcited, no worries: you can pop popcorn in some canola oil and add a variety of low- or no-calorie, sodium-free options to impart flavor. Pair the popcorn with chopped or whole nuts, or toasted sesame seeds or other seeds, to boost your consumption of protein and healthy fats. Or top it with grated Parmesan cheese or cheddar cheese powder, or fold in some dried plums or other dried fruit. Or you can sprinkle small amounts of brown sugar or shredded coconut on the popcorn. You can also use any of the following calorie- and sodium-free options to add some zing to your whole-grain treat: black pepper, cayenne pepper, chili powder, cumin, curry powder, Chinese five-spice powder, fennel seeds, lemon pepper, oregano, red chili flakes, rosemary, sage and thyme. You'll also find a few delicious recipes for popcorn toppers in Chapter 13.

POTATOES

Whether red, white or even a patriotic shade of blue, potatoes rank among the most Vital Foods, and for good reason. Naturally low in fat and sodium and devoid of cholesterol, these starchy vegetables are convenient nutrient-packed additions to your diet. They're delicious and easy to prepare, and they pair well with lean protein, low-fat dairy foods and colorful non-starchy vegetables. And one medium white potato contains only 163 calories.

Sweet Potatoes…Are They Even Potatoes?

According to David Grotto, RD, author of *The Best Things You Can Eat* and *101 Optimal Life Foods,* sweet potatoes are neither potatoes nor yams. He says:

"Technically, to be called a potato, one must be a card-carrying member of the Solanaceae botanical family. Sweet potatoes belong to the Convolvulaceae family, and the word *yam* is derived from the African word *nyami,* which refers to huge root vegetables in the Dioscoreae botanical family. Most Americans who think they have eaten yams have in fact eaten one of four hundred varieties of sweet potatoes instead. True African yams are much starchier and less sweet than the common sweet potato and have white flesh. To avoid confusion in the marketplace, the USDA requires that an additional label of "sweet potato" be placed on anything that is sold as a yam. One thing that is never confusing is just how amazingly delicious and nutritious the sweet potato is. One cup of cooked sweet potatoes supplies over seven times the daily value of vitamin A, is an excellent source of fiber, potassium, vitamin B_6 and vitamin C, and is a good source of pantothenic acid, copper, niacin, thiamine, magnesium, riboflavin and phosphorus."

Among their many virtues, potatoes are replete with complex carbohydrates to boost energy. They also boast fiber—found mostly in their skins—which helps you feel satiated, promotes gastrointestinal health and helps keep your cholesterol levels in check. Potatoes are also a source of resistant starch. Emerging research suggests this fiber-like complex carbohydrate may promote laxation and create so-called "good" bacteria in your gut that help regulate blood sugar and boost fullness, all of which support healthy weight management.

Will Eating Potatoes Make Me Gain Weight?

In a highly publicized 2011 study published in the *New England Journal of Medicine*, Harvard University researchers concluded that having an extra daily serving of potatoes in any form (as potato chips, French fries, or baked, boiled or mashed potatoes) was associated with higher weight gain than other foods and beverages studied. Broken down by potato type, over four years an extra serving of French fries was correlated with a 3.35-pound weight gain; an extra serving of potato chips, with a 1.69-pound weight gain; and an extra serving of baked, boiled or mashed potatoes, with a 0.6-pound weight gain. Although the findings of the study don't prove that eating potatoes specifically causes weight gain, it's no surprise that potato chips and French fries appeared to have more of an impact on body weight than other foods. This is probably because they're higher in calories, fat and salt; they have that can't-have-just-one quality; and eating them is often associated with less healthful habits and a higher calorie intake. The bottom line is prep your potatoes in more healthful ways, and make traditional potato chips or French fries occasional treats instead of a dietary staple.

Potatoes are also notable for their vitamins and minerals. One potato provides an excellent source of vitamin C. A 2007 study published in the *American Journal of Clinical Nutrition* found that vitamin C intake from food sources was linked with a less wrinkled appearance and less age-related skin dryness in middle-aged women. Potatoes also boast high levels of potassium and vitamin B_6, and smaller amounts of other B vitamins, magnesium and phosphorus.

Should You Say No to the Too-Hot Potato?

Many vegetables, including potatoes, contain the amino acid asparagine. When such vegetables are fried, baked or broiled at high temperatures (to make French fries or potato chips, for example), asparagine combines with the sugars in the vegetables to form acrylamide, a chemical linked with cancer in animal studies. Because the National Toxicology Program (NTP), the International Agency for Research on Cancer (IARC), and the United States Environmental Protection Agency (EPA) call acrylamide a "probable human carcinogen," it's wise to boil or microwave whole potatoes with their skins on to avoid acrylamide formation. With a little help from the American Cancer Society, here are some tips to reduce acrylamide formation when you cook potatoes:

Bake more and fry less. Acrylamide formation is highest in fried potatoes, moderate in roasted potato slices and lowest in baked whole potatoes.

Soak 'em. Soak raw potato slices in water for fifteen to thirty minutes, drain and blot before frying or roasting to reduce acrylamide formation.

Store them at room temperature. Instead of refrigerating potatoes, which can raise their sugar levels and subsequently increase acrylamide formation during cooking, store potatoes in a dark, cool place behind closed doors to prevent sprouting.

Cook them quickly. When you bake, roast or fry sliced potatoes, do so for shorter periods of time and at lower temperatures to minimize acrylamide formation. Aim for golden yellow rather than brown potatoes, since a dark color likely means more acrylamide.

Potatoes—especially deeply colored ones—also contain potent chemicals, including carotenoids, anthocyanins, phenolic compounds and chlorogenic acid, that are believed to act as antioxidants, protecting all cells in the human body against free radical damage, which can impair immunity and contribute to heart disease, cancer and other adverse health conditions. Microwaving and baking potatoes tend to minimize antioxidants and nutrient losses more than other cooking methods, like roasting or frying.

Potatoes also are one of the best food sources of kynurenic acid, which arises from the metabolism of the amino acid tryptophan, according to a 2012 study published in *Plant Foods in Human Nutrition*. Researchers believe kynurenic acid—also found in honey—may protect the brain, act as an antioxidant and fight inflammation, which can contribute to disease.

REAL WOMEN COOK-AND EAT-POTATOES!

To maximize the nutrients and taste of potatoes, here are some tips to consider when prepping potatoes (after they're scrubbed) from culinary dietitian Jackie Newgent, RD, author of *1,000 Low-Calorie Recipes:*

- **Hash browns:** Combine diced or sliced unpeeled potatoes with minced shallots, some diced chili pepper and a little olive oil in a skillet. Cover first to steam the vegetables, and then remove the lid, add minced garlic and scallions, and sauté until done. Finish with a handful of minced fresh herbs, including parsley and rosemary.

- **Mashed potatoes:** Keep the potato skins on the potatoes to preserve nutrients and add a homestyle appeal. For creamy moistness, use plain almond milk in place of cow's milk when mashing the potatoes. Also, add roasted garlic for extra flavor (and potential heart health benefits).

- **Baked or microwaved potatoes:** After cooking the potatoes, top them with one pat of butter (but just a pat), a large dollop of plain Greek yogurt or quark (a mild, non-tangy yogurt cheese), and a generous amount of minced fresh chives or scallions. Or add a zing with a dollop of tzatziki dip (a Greek dip made with yogurt, chopped cucumber and mint).

- **Potato salad:** For two pounds of potatoes, use four tablespoons of mayonnaise, three tablespoons of plain Greek yogurt, two tablespoons of stone-ground or Dijon mustard, and one tablespoon of white wine vinegar. Note that two pounds of potatoes serves six.

Vitality Check ✔

Will Potatoes Raise My Blood Sugar?

Although it's true that some potatoes, such as the ever-popular russet potato, have a high glycemic index (GI), white potatoes fall into the medium GI category. But there's no need to bypass even high-GI potatoes. That's because the GI of a single food is likely to be less important when it comes to your blood sugar and your overall health than the glycemic load (GL) of an entire meal. So if you like potatoes, you can reduce their potentially adverse effects on blood sugar by preparing them healthfully, by eating them in small portions (a six-ounce potato or one cup sliced potatoes) and by serving them with lean protein (like fish or chicken) or low-fat dairy.

Starchy Carbs (and a Spoonful of Sugar)

- The Vitality Diet recommends four to five starchy carbs daily, including at least three whole grains.
- Pair starchy carbs (such as oatmeal, whole-grain cereal, quinoa, brown rice, potatoes and popcorn) with other Vital Foods (colorful fruits and vegetables, beans, nuts and seeds, and low-fat dairy) at meals and snack times.
- Emphasize starchy carbs late in the day to promote sound sleep.
- Keep your sugar consumption (table sugar and added sugars found in ready-to-eat cereals and other foods) to no more than 100 to 150 calories daily, and count those calories as Treats (see Chapter 12).

FLIP YOUR FATS AND BOOST OMEGA-3 INTAKE

When you hear the word *fat,* do you immediately associate it with shame, being overweight or weight gain? I'm here to tell you that *fat* is *not* a four-letter word. In fact, whether you're talking about the fat on your hips or thighs or the fat in the foods you eat, embracing your body fat—and incorporating healthy doses of omega-3 fatty acids, found in fish and some plant foods, and monounsaturated fats from nuts, olive oil and avocado—is essential if you want to achieve the 7 Pillars of Vitality. Here are just a few of the ways that body fat and the healthy fats you eat actually help you on your quest to look and feel younger:

- **They fuel you.** Along with carbohydrates and protein, fats provide a key source of energy (calories) for the body. In fact, they're the most concentrated source of energy, because they provide nine calories per gram versus four calories per gram for both carbohydrates and protein. But while your brain and nervous system prefer glucose (sugar) as their main energy source, your muscles increasingly rely on fats for fuel, especially after twenty to thirty minutes of exercise, or when all the glucose in your muscles and liver is used up.

- **They insulate and protect you.** Fats insulate and cushion your entire body, and they guard your brain and vital organs against impact. The layer of fat just beneath the skin's surface acts as a thermostat, regulating body temperature. Fats are also key components of cell membranes—the protective outer layer that holds cells, including those in your skin, together, maintaining their moisture and protecting them against damage caused by the sun and other toxins.

- **They provide brain candy.** You may be surprised to learn that about 60 percent of your brain is made of fatty acids. According to Samantha Heller, MS, RD, author of *Get Smart,* "Fat surrounds each of the 100 billion neurons in the brain to protect, heal and nourish them. It also enables neurons to communicate with one another." Although more data is needed, recent studies suggest that the intake of omega-3 fatty acids may reduce the risk or symptoms of depression and that monounsaturated fat intake may protect against age-related cognitive decline.

- **They help you absorb vitamins.** When you consume vitamins A, D, E and K, collectively known as fat-soluble vitamins, and carotenoids, important antioxidant plant chemicals that produce plants' vibrant color, fats in your diet absorb them and transport them throughout the bloodstream to fatty tissues and the liver, where they're stored for later use.

- **They preserve your youth.** While excess body fat—especially disease-promoting visceral fat, which camps out in your gut—is undesirable, losing too much weight or having too little body fat, especially facial fat, can contribute to a gaunt, unhealthy look. But while many plastic surgeons perform a procedure known as "facial fat grafting," whereby fat from another part of your body is injected into your face to help you look younger, it's much cheaper, and far less painful and dangerous, to consume adequate calories, including those from healthy fats. Having a little extra facial fat can actually improve your overall look.

When you don't consume enough fat in your diet, your body's fat stores can become depleted, and that can lead to menstrual and fertility problems. Too little fat in the diet also can make your skin dry, leave you feeling chilled more often (because you're less insulated) and may make your bones, organs and tissues more vulnerable to injury. But while most of us consume more than enough fat in our daily diets—we get an average of 34 percent of our total daily calories from fat (see Fats: How Much Is Enough? on page 49)—we are out of balance because we overdo saturated and trans-fatty acids while skimping on essential, healthy fats, especially omega-3 fatty acids.

Do 'Em or Ditch 'Em?

Saturated Fatty Acids and Trans-Fatty Acids

Although they provide the body with some structural and physiological support, saturated fatty acids–found abundantly in animal foods, including high-fat meats, butter and full-fat cheese–aren't needed in the diet. The body actually makes enough saturated fat to meet its needs. The high consumption of these foods raises the total blood cholesterol and low-density lipoprotein (LDL) cholesterol (also known as bad cholesterol), which are risk factors for heart disease. Americans consume 11 percent of their total calories in saturated fatty acids. Current guidelines from the American Heart Association call for a daily saturated fatty acid intake of less than 7 percent, and current Dietary Guidelines for Americans recommend an intake of less than 10 percent of total daily calories.

Trans-fatty acids, found naturally in small amounts in animal foods, such as meat and milk products, are also made during hydrogenation–a process that reduces spoilage and rancidity and increases the shelf life of margarines and packaged snacks and desserts. An increased trans-fatty acid intake has been shown to increase LDL cholesterol and decrease good high-density lipoprotein (HDL) cho-lesterol, which can lead to cardiovascular disease. A 2012 study published in *Neurology* also found that a high trans-fatty acid dietary pattern was associated with decreased cognitive function and less total cerebral brain volume (a marker of aging) in older people. Although most experts believe that naturally occurring trans-fatty acids aren't as harmful as artificial ones, it's wise to follow the Institute of Medicine's current recommendations and the Dietary Guidelines for Americans and keep trans-fatty acid intake as low as possible.

Choosing leaner meats, skinless lean poultry, and low-fat and nonfat dairy products, replacing butter and lard with vegetable oils (especially those rich in monounsaturated fat) and avoiding packaged foods that have partially hydrogenated oils in their ingredients lists are just a few of the ways to lower saturated fatty acid and trans-fatty acid intake and still receive the vital benefits fats provide.

Because, gram for gram, fat contains more than twice the calories of either carbohydrates or protein, it's important to be portion savvy when you eat foods that contain fats—even so-called healthy fats—because just a little fat goes a long way. To put it in perspective, one seemingly insignificant tablespoon of olive oil packs about 120 calories—the same number found in almost two cups of raspberries! It's important to be choosy when selecting fatty foods and to keep portions in check to meet, and not exceed, your daily fat needs.

Fats: How Much Is Enough?

According to the Institute of Medicine's Acceptable Macronutrient Distribution Range (AMDR), women should aim for a fat intake of 20 to 35 percent of their total daily calories in order to get the essential nutrients needed and to reduce the risk of chronic diseases, such as cardiovascular disease. For a 1,600-calorie dietary pattern, as outlined in the Vitality Diet (see Chapter 12), that equals 320 to 560 calories, or 36 to 62 grams of fat. Here's what this looks like in terms of food:

36 grams:	**62 grams:**
4 ounces salmon	4 ounces salmon
+ 1 ounce almonds	+ 2 ounces almonds
+ 1 tablespoon olive oil	+ 1 tablespoon olive oil
	+ 1 ounce cheddar cheese

To help you rein in your fat intake and incorporate more unsaturated fat (including omega-3 fatty acids) and less saturated fat and trans fat, the Vitality Diet includes a healthy dose of fish and shellfish, nuts and seeds, and oils. Read on to learn more about these fat-rich foods and how to reap their many benefits (and minimize possible perils).

FISH: A FAR FROM FLAKY CHOICE

From salmon to tuna to shrimp to your favorite sushi, fish and shellfish provide high-quality, filling, muscle-preserving protein with all the amino acids the body needs. They are also low in saturated fats and contain a healthful mix of both monounsaturated fats and polyunsaturated fats. Many types of fish—especially cold-water, oily fish, like salmon, sardines, anchovies, herring and mackerel—are key food sources of two potent long-chain omega-3 fatty acids: eicosapentaenoic acid (EPA) and docosahexaenoic acid (DHA). These essential polyunsaturated fats are integral components in cell membranes and support critical functions in the brain, blood vessels and immune system. EPA creates compounds that help cells divide and grow and also plays a role in blood clotting, muscle activity and digestion, and DHA is critical for brain function. Studies suggest that eating fish has many other vital perks:

- **It helps your ticker tick.** Several studies have linked fish consumption with a reduced risk of coronary heart disease, sudden cardiac death and cerebrovascular disease. According to a 2013 article published in *Food & Function,* a review of three large randomized clinical studies found an inverse association between omega-3 fatty acid intake and cardiovascular disease. In a review that appeared in the *British Medical Journal* in 2012, fish consumption was correlated with a modestly reduced risk of cerebrovascular disease. Researchers believe the benefits were likely due to the interplay of omega-3 fatty acids and other key nutrients found in fish. Another review, this one published in *Current Opinion in Lipidology* in 2012, concluded that eating fatty fish once a week or lean fish twice a week can prevent coronary heart disease.

- **It helps you beat the blues.** In a review published in *Journal of Human Nutrition and Dietetics* in 2013, researchers found that fish consumption was inversely associated with depression risk. In another study, researchers determined that consuming any EPA and DHA from fish was significantly associated with fewer depressive symptoms in more than ten thousand adults. And a prospective study published in the *American Journal of Clinical Nutrition* in 2011 found support for a link between higher intakes of the omega-3 fatty acid alpha-linolenic acid (ALA) and lower intakes of linoleic acid (an omega-6 fatty acid) and a lowered depression risk. In addition to omega-3 fatty acids, the tryptophan content of fish can contribute to the formation of the "feel good" chemical serotonin.

- **It protects your skin.** As both a source of protein, which helps maintain the structure and function of skin, and a source of omega-3 fatty acids, which maintain cell membranes, the feature that provides moisture to and protects skin, fish has been shown to guard against skin cancer. In a prospective study published in the *American Journal of Clinical Nutrition* in 2009, researchers found that the risk of getting precancerous skin lesions decreased by 28 percent among adults who averaged one serving (about 4½ ounces) of oily fish over five days, compared with those who ate oily fish less frequently.

Like all animal foods, fish is a source of dietary cholesterol, and diets high in cholesterol can contribute to an increase in blood cholesterol levels and heart disease, especially if coupled with high saturated fatty acid and trans-fatty acid intake. But consuming a few high-cholesterol options, such as shrimp and lobster, in moderate portions as part of your weekly fish intake won't derail your Vitality Diet, since they are low in saturated fatty acids and provide healthful unsaturated fatty acids and several Vital Nutrients.

Vital Stats: Fish and Shellfish

Here's what you'll find in four ounces (unless otherwise noted) of different types of fish:

Fish Type	Calories	Protein (g)	Total Fat (g)	SFA[1] (g)	MUFA[2] (g)	PUFA[3] (g)	Cholesterol (mg)	Sodium (mg)
Dungeness crab, cooked	125	25	1.4	0.2	2.4	0.5	86	428
Lobster, cooked	101	21.5	1	0.2	0.3	0.4	165	551
Mussels, blue, cooked	195	27	5	1	1.2	1.4	63	418
Oysters, farmed, cooked	90	7.9	2.4	0.8	0.3	0.8	43	185

continued on page 52

Rainbow trout, farmed, cooked	190	27	8.4	1.8	2.7	2	79	69
Salmon coho, farmed, cooked	202	27.5	9.3	2.2	4.1	2.2	71	59
Sardines, drained, canned in oil (3¾ oz)	191	23	10.5	1.5	3.6	4.7	131	465
Shrimp, cooked	135	25.8	1.9	0.6	0.4	0.7	239	1073
Tuna, white, canned in water, drained	145	27	3.8	0.9	0.9	1.3	48	427

1 Saturated fatty acids; **2** Monounsaturated fatty acids; **3** Polyunsaturated fatty acids.

Source: U.S. Department of Agriculture, Agricultural Research Service. 2012. USDA National Nutrient Database for Standard Reference, Release 25. Nutrient Data Laboratory Home Page, www.ars.usda.gov/nutrientdata.

Fish and shellfish provide tons—and I mean tons—of Vital Nutrients. Depending on the type you choose, they are a good or excellent source of several nutrients with vital functions, including vitamin B$_{12}$, niacin, selenium and phosphorus.

Vital Nutrients in Fish and Shellfish

Fish and shellfish offer Good* to Excellent** sources of several vitamins and minerals. Here's how they stack up based on four-ounce portions:

Fish Type	Daily Value	
	Excellent source of:	**Good source of:**
Dungeness crab, cooked	vitamin B$_{12}$, selenium, copper, zinc and niacin	phosphorus, magnesium, riboflavin, potassium and folate
Lobster, cooked	selenium, copper, zinc, vitamin B$_{12}$ and phosphorus	pantothenic acid, magnesium, calcium and niacin
Mussels, blue, cooked	vitamin B$_{12}$, manganese, selenium, iron, phosphorus, riboflavin, vitamin C, thiamin, folate and zinc	niacin, pantothenic acid and magnesium
Oysters, farmed, cooked	vitamin B$_{12}$, zinc, selenium, copper, iron and manganese	phosphorus, vitamin C and niacin
Rainbow trout, farmed, cooked	vitamin D, vitamin B$_{12}$, selenium, niacin, phosphorus, pantothenic acid and vitamin B$_6$	potassium, thiamin and vitamin E
Salmon coho, farmed, cooked	vitamin B$_{12}$, niacin, phosphorus, vitamin B$_6$ and selenium	potassium and pantothenic acid

Sardines, drained, canned in oil (3³⁄₄ oz)	vitamin B_{12}, selenium, phosphorus, vitamin D, calcium and niacin	iron, riboflavin and potassium
Shrimp, cooked	selenium, phosphorus and vitamin B_{12}	niacin, copper, vitamin B_6, zinc, magnesium and calcium
Tuna, white, canned in water, drained	selenium, niacin, phosphorus, vitamin D and vitamin B_{12}	vitamin B_6

*A good source contains 10 to 19 percent of the Daily Value of a nutrient.

**An excellent source contains at least 20 percent of the Daily Value of a nutrient.

Source: U.S. Department of Agriculture, Agricultural Research Service. 2012. USDA National Nutrient Database for Standard Reference, Release 25. Nutrient Data Laboratory Home Page, www.ars.usda.gov/nutrientdata.

(Vitality Check ✔)

What If I Don't Like to Eat Fish?

The Vitality Diet calls for about eight to twelve ounces of fish and shellfish per week to obtain valuable omega-3 fatty acids and other Vital Nutrients. But if you absolutely, positively don't like or won't eat fish, fish oil supplements are an option for filling your omega-3 fatty acid gap. The only catch is that if you choose to take supplements rather than to eat fish, you'll miss out on the other nutrients and beneficial substances in fish that likely work along with omega-3 fatty acids to enhance health. Speak with your doctor before you take any dietary supplement.

NUTS & SEEDS: WHEN GOING NUTS IS A GOOD THING

Besides their great taste and versatility, nuts and seeds are key components in your daily Vitality Diet for so many reasons. Eating nuts and seeds regularly can build a foundation for a healthier diet overall. A study published in *Nutrition Research* in 2012 looked at twenty-four-hour food intake data from national surveys and found that adults who ate at least a quarter ounce of tree nuts daily (these include almonds, Brazil nuts, cashews, hazelnuts, macadamia nuts, pecans, pine nuts, pistachios and walnuts) had higher-quality diets, greater intakes of energy, monounsaturated and polyunsaturated fatty acids, dietary fiber, copper, and magnesium, and lower intakes of carbohydrates, cholesterol and sodium compared with non–nut eaters. In a study that appeared in *Asia Pacific Journal of Clinical Nutrition* in 2010, the same researchers looked at data from thirteen thousand adults and concluded that those who ate at least a quarter ounce of tree nuts daily had a better quality diet, overall, than those who didn't eat tree nuts. They also had higher intakes of fiber, vitamin E, calcium, magnesium, and potassium, and lower sodium intakes.

The perks don't stop there. Studies suggest that eating moderate amounts of nuts and seeds impart vitality-boosting benefits. These include the following:

THEY HELP YOU MANAGE YOUR WEIGHT

In a study published in the *American Journal of Clinical Nutrition* in 2009, researchers evaluated the link between the dietary intake of nuts and weight change over eight years in more than 51,000 twenty- to forty-five-year-old women. They found that women who reported they ate nuts at least twice a week had slightly less than average weight gain than women who reported they rarely ate nuts. When the researchers controlled for lifestyle and other dietary factors, they determined that eating nuts at least twice a week, compared with never or almost never, was associated with a slightly lower risk of weight gain and obesity.

In an article in the *Asia Pacific Journal of Clinical Nutrition* in 2010, researchers suggested that nuts, eaten in moderation, support weight maintainence rather than weight gain, because their calories are inefficiently absorbed. Researchers also noted that nuts promote satiety (the feeling of fullness) and help the body burn more calories at rest and during digestion. Finally, they suggested that including nuts as part of a weight-loss regimen can lead to better compliance and greater weight loss compared with regimens that do not include nuts.

THEY KEEP YOUR HEART HEALTHY AND WARD OFF DISEASE

Nuts received a high honor in 2003 from the Food and Drug Administration (FDA) when it approved the first qualified health claim for food for use on package labels. It reads, "Scientific evidence suggests but does not prove that eating 1.5 ounces per day of most nuts, as part of a diet low in saturated fat and cholesterol, may reduce the risk of heart disease." And the supportive studies keep pouring in:

- In a review published in the *Journal of Nutrition* in 2005, researchers found that eating fifty to one hundred grams (about 1.8 to 3.5 ounces) of nuts, such as almonds, pecans, or walnuts, five or more times a week as part of a heart-healthy, moderate-fat diet (where fat is about 35 percent of total calories) significantly lowered total cholesterol and LDL cholesterol in adults with and without hypertension, compared with control diets without nuts. Similarly, the consumption of tree nuts was shown to reduce LDL cholesterol by 3 to 19 percent when compared to following Western and lower-fat diets in a 2006 study published in the *British Journal of Nutrition*.

- In a review published in the *British Journal of Nutrition* in 2006, researchers analyzed several studies and determined that the risk of coronary heart disease (CHD) was 37 percent lower for those consuming nuts more than four times per week compared to those who never or seldom consumed nuts. Each weekly serving of nuts was also estimated to reduce CHD risk by 8.3 percent.

- A six-year study that appeared in *Public Health Nutrition* in 2012 found that adults who ate at least two weekly servings of nuts had a 32 percent lower risk of developing metabolic syndrome—a cluster of symptoms that contributes to both cardiovascular disease and type 2 diabetes—than those who seldom or never ate nuts.

- A study in the *Journal of the American College of Nutrition* in 2011 found that consuming at least a quarter ounce of nuts daily was associated with decreased body mass index, waist circumference and systolic blood pressure—risk factors for cardiovascular disease, type 2 diabetes and metabolic syndrome. Adults who ate tree nuts also had a lower body weight than non–nut eaters.

- According to an article published in *Current Atherosclerosis Report* in 2010, there's emerging evidence that in addition to their heart-health benefits, nuts may play a role in reducing oxidative stress and inflammation.

THEY PROVIDE NUTRIENTS

Although it's true that nuts and seeds deliver a mix of fats in a hearty dose, most of the fat in most types of nuts is monounsaturated fat, the type that can reduce blood cholesterol levels and lower heart disease and stroke risk, especially when consumed in place of saturated fat and trans-fatty acids. (Most nuts are low in artery-clogging saturated fat and contain no cholesterol.) Nuts are also a source of polyunsaturated fatty acids, including linoleic acid and omega-3 fatty acids—essential fats that need to be included in our diets since our bodies cannot manufacture them. Walnuts, chia seeds and flaxseeds also provide omega-3 polyunsaturated fatty acids called alpha-linolenic acid (ALA). Although there's limited evidence about the health benefits of ALA, a small fraction of ALA is converted in the body into EPA and DHA, the potent omega-3 fatty acids found in fish. Nuts and seeds also boost protein and fiber to fill you up. And even though salted nuts taste salty, most brands of nuts don't have much added salt, since it's only on the surface, right there for the tasting!

Vital Stats: Nuts and Seeds

Here's what you'll find in one ounce of unsalted nuts and seeds:

Type/Portion[1]	Calories	Total Fat (g)	MUFA[2] (g)	PUFA[3] (g)	SFA[4] (g)	Protein (g)	Fiber (g)
Almonds (24)	169	14.8	9.2	3.7	1.1	6	3.1
Brazil nuts (6)	186	18.8	7.0	5.8	4.3	4.1	2.1
Cashews (18)	163	13	7.7	2.2	2.6	4.3	0.9
Chia seeds (3 tbsp)	138	8.7	0.7	6.7	0.9	4.7	9.8
Flaxseed (4 tbsp, ground)	150	12	2.1	8	1	5.1	7.6
Hazelnuts (20)	183	18	13.2	2.4	1.3	4.3	2.7
Macadamia nuts (10-12)	204	22	16.8	0.4	3.4	2.2	2.3
Peanuts* (28)	166	14	7	4.4	2	6.7	0.1

Pecans (10 whole, 20 halves)	201	21	12.4	5.8	1.8	2.7	2.7
Pistachios (49)	161	12.7	6.7	3.8	1.5	5.9	0.1
Sunflower seeds (4 tbsp)	165	14	2.7	9.3	1.5	5.5	3.1
Walnuts, English (7 whole, 14 halves)	185	18.5	2.5	13.4	1.7	4.3	1.9

1 These are approximate portions; **2** Monounsaturated fatty acids; **3** Polyunsaturated fatty acids; **4** Saturated fatty acids.

*Peanuts are technically legumes but have a similar nutritional profile to nuts and seeds and are eaten like them.

Source: U.S. Department of Agriculture, Agricultural Research Service. 2012. USDA National Nutrient Database for Standard Reference, Release 25. Nutrient Data Laboratory Home Page, www.ars.usda.gov/nutrientdata.

Collectively, nuts and seeds are good or excellent sources of several vitamins and minerals (see Glossary for more about these Vital Nutrients). Here's how they stack up based on one-ounce portions:

- **Almonds** are a good source of riboflavin, copper and phosphorus and an excellent source of vitamin E, manganese and magnesium.

- **Brazil nuts** are a good source of manganese and thiamine and an excellent source of selenium, magnesium, copper and phosphorus.

- **Cashews** are a good source of magnesium, phosphorus, vitamin K, manganese and zinc and an excellent source of copper.

- **Chia seeds** are a good source of calcium, copper, niacin and iron and an excellent source of thiamine, manganese, phosphorus, magnesium and selenium.

- **English walnuts** are a good source of pantothenic acid and magnesium and an excellent source of manganese and copper.

- **Flaxseeds** are a good source of phosphorus, copper and selenium and an excellent source of manganese, thiamine and magnesium.

- **Hazelnuts** are a good source of vitamin E and magnesium and an excellent source of manganese and copper.

- **Macadamia nuts** are a good source of thiamine and an excellent source of manganese.

- **Peanuts** are a good source of niacin, magnesium, folate and phosphorus and an excellent source of manganese.

- **Pecans** are a good source of copper and an excellent source of manganese.

- **Pine nuts** are a good source of vitamin K, copper, magnesium, phosphorus and zinc and an excellent source of manganese.

- **Pistachios** are a good source of copper, manganese, vitamin B_6, phosphorus and thiamine.

- **Sunflower seeds** are a good source of pantothenic acid, folate, vitamin B_6 and zinc and an excellent source of phosphorus, selenium, manganese, copper and vitamin E.

Nuts and seeds also possess an array of powerful plant chemicals that have antioxidant and other properties. According to a review published in *Nutrition Research Reviews* in 2011, tree nuts contain plant chemicals, including carotenoids, phenolic acids, phytosterols and polyphenolic compounds (such as flavonoids, proanthocyanidins and stilbenes) that have antioxidant, anti-inflammatory and other protective benefits. An extensive review of antioxidants in food published in *Nutrition Journal* in 2010 also showed higher levels in nuts with pellicles (the thin skins or films that surround some nuts) than in those without.

Vitality Check ✓

Should You Go Nuts for Nut Butters?

If you like to eat peanut butter or other nut butters by the spoonful, you'll get a similar mix of healthy fats, protein, vitamins, minerals and antioxidants that you'd find in nuts. But you'll also find some added sugar and a lot more sodium—and sometimes even extra oil, such as cottonseed oil (which is high in saturated fat). Also, reduced-fat nut butters may not be a nutritional bargain. They typically have about the same number of calories as full-fat options, and what they lack in fat, they make up for in added sugar, like corn syrup solids or molasses. Brands vary a lot, so be sure to read Nutrition Facts panels and ingredients lists on labels, and look for those made with little added sugar and sodium. A few of my favorite options are Trader Joe's Organic Peanut Butter, Kraft All-Natural Peanut Butter and Earth Balance Natural Peanut Butter. But be aware that nut butters may not be an even nutritional swap for unsalted raw or dry-roasted nuts.

OILS FOR A HEALTHY HEART

Although not technically foods, oils (fats that are liquid at room temperature) are an integral component of the Vitality Diet because of the contributions they make not only to the taste, texture and appeal of meals, but also to nutrient intake. They are found in fish, nuts and seeds, as discussed previously, and also in such foods as avocados and olives (see Chapter 8). Olive oil, canola oil and other vegetable oils are used to cook and flavor foods. These oils are rich in monounsaturated and polyunsaturated fats (including essential fats)—fats that don't raise LDL (bad) cholesterol levels. When used in place of foods rich in saturated fatty acids (butter and sour cream, for example) and trans-fatty acids (found in some margarines and spreads), oils can help lower cholesterol levels and reduce heart disease risk. Many oils are a significant dietary source of vitamin E, an important fat-soluble vitamin that acts as an antioxidant and maintains immune cell function.

Many oils contain a mix of fats. Those that have a high proportion of monounsaturated fat include safflower oil, olive oil, canola oil, peanut oil, soybean oil and sesame oil. Among those with a high proportion of polyunsaturated fat are corn oil, cottonseed oil, flaxseed oil, soybean oil, sunflower oil and walnut oil. And flaxseed oil is particularly rich in the omega-3 fatty acid ALA.

Vital Stats: Oils

Here's what you'll find in 1 teaspoon of oil:

Oil	Calories	Total Fat (g)	MUFA[1] (g)	PUFA[2] (g)	SFA[3] (g)
Canola oil*	40	4.5	2.9	1.3	0.3
Corn oil	40	4.5	1.3	2.5	0.6
Cottonseed oil	40	4.5	0.8	2.3	1.2
Flaxseed oil*	40	4.5	0.8	3.1	0.1
Olive oil	40	4.5	3.3	0.5	0.6
Peanut oil	40	4.5	2.1	1.4	0.8

continued on page 60

Safflower oil	40	4.5	3.4	0.6	0.3
Sesame oil	40	4.5	1.8	1.9	0.6
Soybean oil*	40	4.5	1	2.6	0.7
Sunflower oil	40	4.5	0.88	2.96	0.46
Walnut oil*	40	4.5	1	2.9	0.41

*These oils also contain the omega-3 fatty acid ALA, though flaxseed oil has the highest concentration of ALA among these oils. **1** Monounsaturated fatty acids; **2** Polyunsaturated fatty acids; **3** Saturated fatty acids.

Source: U.S. Department of Agriculture, Agricultural Research Service. 2012. USDA National Nutrient Database for Standard Reference, Release 25. Nutrient Data Laboratory Home Page, www.ars.usda.gov/nutrientdata.

BALANCING HEALTHY FATS

Even though the American Heart Association and current Dietary Guidelines for Americans recommend consuming a diet rich in monounsaturated and polyunsaturated fatty acids from oils and other foods naturally rich in these nutrients in the context of a diet low in saturated and trans-fatty acids, emerging research suggests that we need to pay more attention to the balance between omega-3 fatty acids and omega-6 fatty acids in our diets and essentially *flip our fats*. In an article published in *Experimental Biology and Medicine* in 2008, researchers noted that while humans may have evolved on a diet with equal parts omega-6 and omega-3 fatty acids, Western diets currently provide excessive amounts of omega-6 fatty acids and deficient amounts of omega-3 fatty acids. The researchers suggest that this imbalance can increase the risk of cardiovascular disease, cancer, and inflammatory and autoimmune diseases. A study of older people published in *Psychosomatic Medicine* in 2007 also found that diets with high omega-6: omega-3 ratios were associated with increased depression and inflammation owing to the increased production of substances called pro-inflammatory cytokines. Other studies show that omega-6 fatty acids can interfere with the synthesis of serotonin and other brain chemicals and adversely impact behavior, mood and sleep.

Coconut Oil: Is It All That It's Cracked Up to Be?

Want to know the real deal about coconut oil? See what the very sensible Janet Helm, MS, RD, writer of the blog *Nutrition Unplugged* and author of *The Food Lover's Healthy Habits Cookbook,* has to say: Coconut oil is enjoying its day in the sun, heavily promoted on websites and extolled by certain experts who claim this "miraculous" tropical oil can prevent or cure ailments ranging from heart disease and cancer to Alzheimer's disease. Coconut oil enthusiasts also say this elixir oil can help you lose weight, yet gobbling up the recommended three to five tablespoons of coconut oil a day would add up to six hundred calories. Not such a smart strategy to me. So how did all of this get started? Many of the sites that promote and sell coconut oil (including jars of virgin coconut oil and coconut oil supplements) originate from coconut-producing countries—including India, Indonesia and the Philippines. Many of the arguments made by these companies are related to the low rates of heart disease in tropical populations that have consumed large quantities of coconut oil for centuries. Yet, that's not reliable evidence, since other diet and lifestyle factors play a larger role. Coconut oil is the most saturated of all fats—including butter. It's true that the type of saturated fat in coconut oil may not raise blood cholesterol levels the same as other saturated fats. But there's no scientific evidence that the fat has any protective effects. One recent study found that coconut oil raised LDL or "bad" cholesterol. Even if it's neutral, there's no reason to guzzle it up by the spoonful. The structure of coconut oil is different than other oils because it contains a high percentage of medium-chain triglycerides, or MCTs. That means we metabolize coconut oil a bit differently compared to oils with mostly long-chain triglycerides. Yet, this does not give coconut oil super powers to melt fat. There's just no convincing evidence that adding coconut oil will help you lose weight or improve your health. If you like the taste, it's fine to use it occasionally in cooking or in baking (as a substitute for butter or shortening). It's not a good idea, however, to make a full switch. You'll not only add more saturated fats to your diet, but you'll miss out on all the well-documented benefits of olive, canola and other liquid oils.

Although much more data is needed, it's prudent to consume small amounts of vegetable oils and to emphasize those that are rich in monounsaturated fat and omega-3 fatty acids (in the form of ALA) as part of your Vitality Diet. While it's perfectly fine to have other fatty oils or add-ons, such as coconut oil (see Coconut Oil: Is It All That It's Cracked Up to Be?), butter, sour cream or cream cheese, they are high in saturated fat, so they'll count as treats in the Vitality Diet (see Chapter 12).

Healthy Fats

- Aim for about four to five servings of healthy fats daily. To meet that goal, consume at least two portions of nuts, nut butters and seeds* daily.
- Choose foods that are rich in healthy fats, such as fatty fish, which has an abundance of omega-3 fatty acids, and nuts/seeds, which are an excellent source of monounsaturated and polyunsaturated fatty acids.
- Choose oils that are high in mostly unsaturated fats, especially monounsaturated fatty acids, such as olive oil, canola oil and safflower oil.
- Choose meats and other animal foods that are lower in saturated fat.

*Nuts, nut butters and seeds also count as proteins. See Chapters 5 and 12.

EMPOWER YOURSELF WITH PROTEIN

Protein is a vital component of the body—and of the Vitality Diet. While it provides a source of energy, just like carbohydrates and fat, protein has many unique roles. Found in virtually every body part, protein is a nutrient that literally keeps your body intact and enables you to perform countless activities with vim and vigor—and to look and feel your best while doing them! Although you don't want to overdose on protein-rich foods, having "just enough" as part of your Vitality Diet can do wonders to protect you from the ravages of aging.

VITAL ROLES OF PROTEIN

Protein is good for your body in so many ways. It:

- **Gives your body structure.** For example, collagen—the body's most abundant protein—protects and supports the structure and function of skin, bones, muscles, tendons, ligaments and cartilage. And keratin is a protein that forms the protective outer layer of skin and provides structure for hair and nails.

- **Delivers oxygen throughout the body.** Hemoglobin, a protein found mainly in the bloodstream, plays a key role in respiration by delivering much-needed oxygen to nearly every body part, including muscles, bones and organs.

- **Helps you digest food.** Enzymes are proteins found in your saliva, stomach, pancreas and small intestine. They support vital chemical reactions, including digestion—the breakdown of food so it can be absorbed and used by the body.

- **Helps regulate blood sugar levels.** Insulin and glucagon are protein-based peptide hormones that play an integral role in keeping levels of glucose—the body's main energy source—steady in the blood.

- **Fills you up.** Studies suggest that protein fills you up and is more satiating than either carbohydrate or fat.

- **Makes you move.** Actin and myosin are proteins that help muscles contract, enabling you to breathe, blink, walk, ride a bike and dance.

- **Protects against infection and illness.** Antibodies are proteins created by the immune system to defend the body against invaders, such as bacteria or viruses.

IT GIVES YOUR BRAIN A BOOST

Dietary protein also provides your body with amino acids. Some create important brain chemicals, called neurotransmitters, which have a direct impact on how you feel and how you respond to daily and chronic stressors. For example, the amino acid tryptophan makes serotonin, a neurotransmitter believed to play a role in regulating mood, appetite and sleep. Tyrosine, another amino acid, creates the neurotransmitters norepinephrine (noradrenaline) and epinephrine (adrenaline)—also known as stress hormones—which arouse the body and make it ready for action, as well as dopamine, which is associated with pleasure and pain.

IT'S A BOON FOR YOUR MUSCLES AND BONES

If you're not yet convinced that dietary protein can help you shine, this should seal the deal: consuming enough protein can, to at least some extent, protect your muscles and bones from aging. Eating protein in small doses throughout the day, especially if you're a regular exerciser, can help you build muscle or at least avoid slow and steady muscle loss, which is experienced by many women in their forties (and younger, for those who don't stay active).

Having enough protein is not only crucial for maintaining muscle mass, but also for keeping your metabolism revved up while you cut calories to lose weight. When your diet lacks adequate protein, you lose vital muscle along with some body fat, which will cause your metabolism—and you—to slow down to conserve energy. That's not exactly a winning recipe for looking and feeling strong, fit and lean, is it? And when it comes to bones, while most women can preserve bone health well into their thirties and forties, once menopause hits, your bones start to degrade at a rapid rate. That's why arming yourself now with a diet that provides adequate—but not excessive—protein can reduce your risk of weak or broken bones (in part by enhancing calcium absorption), a condition that may undermine your otherwise vibrant life. There's also evidence that eating adequate protein while you cut calories to lose weight can protect your bones, not just your muscles.

PROTEIN 101

When you consume dietary protein—whether from fish, a burger, a handful of nuts or a cup of yogurt—the protein is broken down into as many as twenty different amino acids, often referred to as the "building blocks" of protein. These amino acids are linked in countless ways to create tens of thousands of unique proteins that help the body function. Eleven amino acids are naturally made by the body to meet its needs, but nine of them can't be made at all—or in enough quantity—so it's critical to get these "essential" amino acids from your diet by eating a variety of protein-rich foods. Animal foods, such as fish, poultry, lean meat, eggs and dairy products, are considered high-quality protein sources since they contain all the essential amino acids. Plant foods, such as beans and peas, nuts, nut butters and seeds and, to a lesser extent, grains and vegetables, are also rich in amino acids, but only a handful, such as soybeans, quinoa and spinach, are considered high-quality protein since they naturally contain all the essential amino acids. Although the Vitality Diet includes animal sources of protein, if you don't consume these foods, you can still meet your protein and essential amino acids needs—and get that much closer to achieving the 7 Pillars of Vitality—by incorporating protein-packed plant foods into your meals each and every day.

HOW MUCH IS ENOUGH?

There are a few ways dietitians help clients figure out their daily protein needs. Based on the Recommended Dietary Allowance (RDA), a typical woman between the ages of nineteen and seventy requires 0.8 grams/kilogram body weight of protein each day. For a woman who weighs 120 pounds, that's 44 grams (the amount you'd find in four ounces of salmon, one egg, a quarter cup of lentils and two ounces of tofu). The RDA for a woman who weighs 160 pounds is 58 grams (the amount you'd find in four ounces of salmon, one egg, a quarter cup of lentils and two ounces of tofu plus a cup of nonfat yogurt). Some experts recommend a higher RDA of protein for adults to prevent the muscle loss that occurs with aging.

Another tool to determine protein needs—and one that considers the total diet and the number of calories people consume based on their weight, height, activity level, body frame and other variables—is the Institute of Medicine's Acceptable Macronutrient Distribution Range (AMDR). According to this formula, your protein intake should be about 10 to 35 percent of your total daily calories. So, if you consume about 1,600 calories per day (see Chapter 12 for guidelines), that's between 160 calories (40 grams) and 560 calories (140 grams) of protein. Using the RDA and the AMDR together, your daily protein intake should be between 58 grams and 140 grams. As long as you are also meeting the other AMDR (and Vitality Diet) recommendations for carbohydrates and fat (as discussed in Chapters 3 and 4, respectively), you're likely meeting your basic nutrient needs.

A High-Protein Diet

For years, many dieters have ramped up their intake of protein-rich foods, often at the expense of carbohydrate-rich foods, to lose weight, but is this a smart, safe strategy? A comprehensive review published in the *European Journal of Clinical Nutrition* in 2011 assessed thirty-eight randomized, controlled trials comparing the effects of higher- and lower-protein diets on body weight. Researchers found moderate evidence that higher-protein diets resulted in greater weight loss, a greater decrease in body mass index and a greater reduction in waist circumference than lower-protein diets. The authors noted that diets emphasizing modest, instead of large, increases in protein intake were more likely to have an ameliorative effect on body mass index and other disease factors. Although more long-term data is needed, the authors concluded that the beneficial effects of a higher-protein diet on weight loss were small and should be weighed against the potential negative gastrointestinal effects (such as constipation, halitosis, diarrhea, bloating and fullness) and other adverse effects of higher-protein diets that have been reported in some studies. The bottom line? Ditch the high-protein diet and opt instead for a diet that's moderate in protein and fat. Balance that out with about half of your total calories from carbohydrates, in keeping with the Vitality Diet (see Chapter 12).

In the following pages, you'll learn more about some of my favorite Vital Foods that are good sources of protein, including eggs, poultry and lean beef, beans and peas, and soy foods. Other protein sources, such as fish, shellfish and dairy foods, are covered extensively in Chapters 4 and Chapter 7, respectively.

EGGS

While many women think eggs are incredible, some find them inedible. Wherever you stand when it comes to eggs (I personally love them), no one can deny that they boast an excellent assortment of nutrients and other beneficial substances, making them key components of a Vitality Diet.

ON THE SUNNY SIDE

With only seventy-two calories in a large one, eggs are a great source of high-quality protein. They also contain heart-healthy monounsaturated and polyunsaturated fatty acids and are relatively low in sodium. One whole egg is an excellent source of selenium and a good source of riboflavin and vitamin D. Eggs also contains sulfur (especially in the yolks) and choline (see the Glossary to learn more about these Vital Nutrients).

In addition, egg yolks contain some lutein and zeaxanthan—carotenoid antioxidants that may reduce the risk of age-related macular degeneration and cataracts, and protect against heart disease, stroke and some cancers. Having one egg a day for five weeks was shown to significantly increase blood levels of these antioxidants without adversely affecting blood cholesterol levels in a small study of older adults published in the *Journal of Nutrition* in 2006.

POSSIBLE PERILS

Despite their many virtues, eggs are also a source of saturated fat. But while diets high in saturated fat can raise total cholesterol and LDL (bad) cholesterol—risk factors for cardiovascular disease—only one-third of the fat in eggs is saturated. The remainder is heart-healthy monounsaturated and polyunsaturated fat. Although eggs are also notorious for the amount of cholesterol they contain, several studies have questioned the link between dietary cholesterol and heart disease and stroke. In a 2003 study that appeared in the *British Medical Journal,* Harvard researchers followed 115,000 adults for fourteen years and found that eating an egg a day was not associated with an increased risk of coronary heart disease and stroke. Several other recent clinical trials have also failed to show adverse effects of long-term egg consumption on blood cholesterol and other measures of cardiovascular health. Still, many experts urge a limited intake of dietary cholesterol from egg yolks and other sources, especially for adults with, or at risk for, cardiovascular disease. Although current federal dietary guidelines call for fewer than three hundred milligrams of cholesterol daily, the American Heart Association (AHA) and the National Cholesterol Education Program (NCEP) recommend fewer than two hundred milligrams for those with heart disease, type 2 diabetes or high LDL (bad) cholesterol levels.

Can Eating Eggs = Eating Less?

We know that eggs are packed with high-quality protein, which helps you feel full longer and stay energized, but there's also evidence that they may even help you eat less–a bonus if you're trying to cut your calorie intake. In one study published in the *European Journal of Nutrition* in 2012, thirty healthy men were randomly assigned to eat one of three test breakfasts–eggs on toast, cornflakes with milk and toast, or a croissant and orange juice–on three separate occasions, each separated by one week. Subjects felt more full and less hungry and had less desire to eat after the egg breakfast than the other breakfasts. They also ate less at lunch and dinner after having the egg breakfast as opposed to the other breakfasts. In an earlier study published in *Nutrition Research* in 2010, men were given an egg breakfast or a bagel breakfast in random order separated by a week. When given eggs for breakfast, they were more satisfied three hours later, and they consumed fewer calories over the next twenty-four hours compared with when they ate the bagel breakfast. And in a study that appeared in the *International Journal of Food Science Nutrition* in 2011, adults ate three test lunches–an omelet, a skinless potato or a chicken sandwich (each with same calorie load)–following a standard breakfast. Researchers found that the egg lunch was significantly more satisfying than the potato lunch, and they concluded that having eggs at lunch could increase satiety more than a carbohydrate meal and may even help reduce calorie intake between meals.

So, if you like eggs, what's stopping you? If you're healthy, there's no reason why you can't have up to one whole egg a day (or about seven a week). Just remember, eggs are ingredients in so many prepared foods, including baked goods, French toast, some salad dressings (like Caesar), meatballs and meat loaf. If you have high cholesterol, heart disease or type 2 diabetes, you may want to cut back more on eggs and other animal foods rich in saturated fat and cholesterol. And if you opt for egg whites only, you'll lose three-quarters of the calories and all the cholesterol and saturated fat. But be mindful that you'll also forfeit all the healthy fats, some protein, and all the choline, lutein and zeaxanthin. Opting for half whole eggs and half egg whites might be a smarter bet.

BEANS AND PEAS

Dried peas, lentils, chickpeas and beans, also known as pulses, are at the heart of the Vitality Diet. These mature, edible seeds of legumes overflow with nutrients and powerful plant chemicals, which together help you move toward achieving the 7 Pillars of Vitality in more ways than one. There's evidence that eating legumes can improve your diet and overall health, and may even help you live longer. A study published in the *Journal of the American Dietetic Association* in 2009 showed that those who consumed a half cup of dried beans and peas daily had higher intakes of fiber, protein, folate, zinc, iron and magnesium, and had lower intakes of total fat and saturated fat, when compared with non–pulse eaters. In another study, this one published in the *Journal of the American College of Nutrition* in 2008, adults who consumed beans had higher intakes of dietary fiber, potassium, magnesium, iron and copper; lower systolic blood pressure; lower body weight; a smaller waist circumference; and a lower risk of being obese than those who didn't eat beans. And in the "Food Habits in Later Life" study, a worldwide seven-year study of 785 adults aged seventy and above, Australian researchers found that legume consumption predicted longevity better than any other dietary component.

DYNAMIC DUO FOR YOUR HEALTH

So, what exactly is it about beans that makes them such dietary assets? Besides being rich protein sources, about two-thirds of their calories come from complex carbohydrates, mainly in the form of resistant starch. Unlike most starches, which are digested and absorbed in the small intestine, resistant starch behaves like dietary fiber, resisting digestion in the small intestine and going to the large intestine, where it's slowly fermented. Although more research is needed, emerging studies suggest that consuming resistant starch may help improve glucose and insulin responses to a meal, may reduce cholesterol and triglyceride levels, and may play a role in satiety and weight management. Beans and peas are also great sources of both soluble and insoluble fiber. Furthermore, beans have little fat and no cholesterol, and dried varieties are naturally low in sodium. Beans also have low glycemic index values and have little impact on blood sugar levels. And because they're gluten-free, they're safe (and tasty) dietary additions for those with celiac disease or gluten intolerance. (See Vital Stats: Beans and Peas on page 71.)

Vital Stats: Beans and Peas

Here's how your favorite beans and peas measure up when it comes to nutrition. All values are for $^1/_4$ cup (1 Beans/Peas in The Vitality Diet, see Chapter 12):

	Calories	Protein (g)	Total Fat (g)	Carbohydrate (g)	Fiber (g)	Sodium (mg)	Daily Values*
Black beans, canned	55	3.62	<1	10	4.1	230	Good source of fiber
Black beans, cooked	57	3.81	<1	10.2	3.7	0	Good source of fiber and folate
Black eyed peas, canned	46	2.8	<1	8	2	179	N/A[1]
Black eyed peas, cooked	50	3.3	<1	9	2.8	2	Excellent source of folate; Good source of fiber and manganese
Chickpeas, canned, (mature seeds)	52	2.7	1	8.7	2.7	81	Good source of manganese
Chickpeas, cooked	67	3.6	1	11	3.1	3	Excellent source of manganese; Good source of fiber and folate
Green peas, canned	29	1.9	<1	5.4	1.7	1	Excellent source of niacin
Green peas, cooked	34	2	<1	6.3	2.2	1	Good source of vitamin K and manganese
Kidney beans, canned	52	3.3	<1	9.3	3.4	189	Good source of fiber
Kidney beans, cooked	56	3.8	<1	10	2.8	0	Good source of fiber and folate
Lentils, mature seeds, cooked	57	4.5	<1	10	3.9	1	Excellent source of folate; Good source of fiber and manganese
Lima beans, canned	48	3	<1	9	3	0	Good source of fiber and manganese
Lima beans, cooked	54	3.7	<1	9.8	3.3	1	Good source of fiber and manganese

continued on page 72

	Calories	Protein (g)	Total Fat (g)	Carbohydrate (g)	Fiber (g)	Sodium (mg)	Daily Values*
Pinto beans, canned	49	3	<1	8.8	2.3	90	N/A[1]
Pinto beans, cooked	61	3.9	<1	11	3.8	0	Good source of fiber and folate
Split peas, cooked	58	4	<1	10	4.1	1	Good source of fiber
White beans, canned	75	4.8	<1	14	3	0	Good source of fiber, manganese, iron, and folate
White beans, cooked	62	4.4	<1	11.22	2.8	0	Good source of fiber and manganese

1 Not applicable.

*An excellent source means the food contains at least 20 percent of the Daily Value of a nutrient; a good source means the food contains 10 to 19 percent of the Daily value of a nutrient.

Source: U.S. Department of Agriculture, Agricultural Research Service. 2012. USDA National Nutrient Database for Standard Reference, Release 25. Nutrient Data Laboratory Home Page, www.ars.usda.gov/ba/bhnrc/ndi.

One quarter cup of beans or peas is a good or excellent source of nutrients, including fiber, folate and manganese, and has smaller amounts of vitamins and minerals, such as vitamin C, thiamine, phosphorous, iron and magnesium.

Dried peas, lentils, chickpeas and beans are also rich sources of polyphenols, phytosterols and other phytochemicals, many of which act as antioxidants, protecting body cells from free-radical damage.

BEANS, BEANS, THEY'RE GOOD FOR YOUR HEART

You've no doubt heard this expression, and studies suggest that beans can benefit your heart by lowering blood cholesterol levels and reducing your risk for heart disease and heart attack. In a study published in the *British Journal of Nutrition* in 2012, adults aged fifty and older who consumed a pulse-based diet featuring two daily ¾-cup servings of beans, chickpeas, peas or lentils experienced significant reductions in total cholesterol and LDL (bad) cholesterol. In a review in *Nutrition, Metabolism and Cardiovascular*

Disease in 2011, researchers looked at ten studies conducted with 265 adults and found that adherence to a diet rich in non-soy legumes, such as chickpeas, pinto beans, canned baked beans, peas and navy beans, led to a decrease in total cholesterol and LDL (bad) cholesterol. Researchers speculated that the positive effects were likely due to the fiber in legumes (including soluble fiber) and the phytochemicals (such as phytosterols) they contain.

THE REAL DEAL VERSUS DIABETES

Consuming beans and peas may also lower the risk of type 2 diabetes or help in the management of the disease, in large part because of their low glycemic index. In a review article published in the *British Nutrition Journal* in 2012, researchers determined that eating more beans, such as pinto, black, navy or kidney beans, appeared to be particularly beneficial in preventing and treating conditions that result from increased glycemic stress (hyperglycemia and hyperinsulinemia), such as type 2 diabetes. Another review article, this one of forty-one studies, published in *Diabetologia* in 2009, found that consuming pulses either alone or as part of a low glycemic index or a high-fiber diet promoted long-term glycemic control, which is essential for the prevention and management of diabetes.

OTHER BEAN BENEFITS

Although there's not enough proof to assert that eating beans will benefit your waistline or your weight, their unique combination of complex carbohydrates (including resistant starch), protein and fiber may help you lose weight, better manage your weight or prevent weight gain, especially if they're consumed in place of animal-protein foods, such as fatty meats and poultry and fried fish.

Beans may also help your body fight cancer. According to Karen Collins, MS, RD, nutrition advisor for the American Institute for Cancer Research, "Beans are rich in phytochemicals that can provide antioxidant protection against DNA damage and fight inflammation. They're also an important source of fiber (especially soluble fiber) that can decrease the risk of colorectal cancer and offer modest reduction in breast cancer risk." Collins adds, "Healthy bacteria in our gut use dietary fiber and resistant starch (abundant in dried beans) to produce butyrate, a fatty acid that seems to protect colon cells."

There's also some evidence that eating beans may benefit your mood and your brain health. A study in *Public Health Nutrition* in 2010 found that a moderate intake of legumes (one to two servings weekly) protected women going through menopause against severely depressed moods. And a study published in the *Journal of Nutrition, Health and Aging* in 2012 concluded that the low consumption of legumes and vegetables was correlated with cognitive decline in older Chinese adults.

HOW TO SLIP 'EM IN

The Vitality Diet calls for at least 1½ cups of dried peas, lentils, chickpeas and beans each week, consistent with current federal dietary guidelines. Unfortunately, most of us consume far less. In fact, a 2009 study published in the *Journal of the American Dietetic Association* found that only 7.9 percent of adults consume dried beans and peas on any given day. Here are seven ways to seamlessly slip beans and peas into your Vitality Diet from registered dietitian (and bean lover) Andrea Giancoli, MPH, RD:

- **Add them to salads.** Pair kidney beans, black beans, garbanzo beans or peas with salad greens; mix together diced avocado, corn and pinto beans or black beans and season with lemon juice or rice vinegar to make a side salad (this is also great as a dip with corn tortilla chips); enjoy a lentil salad made with lentils, parsley, cucumber, green onions, lemon juice and olive oil (if desired); make an entrée salad by combining canned tuna, cannellini beans, diced tomatoes and diced onions with a little olive oil; or make a pasta salad with beans.

- **Serve them Mexican style.** Have vegetarian non-refried pinto beans on their own, topped with guacamole, in a tostada or as a side dish with fish tacos or spinach enchiladas; use black beans or pinto beans to make vegetarian tacos; or mix beans with ground beef for a fiber-filled taco.

- **Stir them into soup.** For a hearty starter or main dish, try pureed black bean soup or navy bean soup; vegetarian split pea soup (like Andersen's); or lentil soup cooked with celery, carrots and bay leaves.

- **Do a dip (or a dollop).** Dip carrots and whole-wheat crackers (Original Triscuits or Triscuit Thin Crisps) in hummus made with garbanzo or cannellini beans; use hummus (or any mashed beans) as a sandwich spread instead of mayonnaise; or make your own dip by pureeing your favorite beans and adding minced cilantro, minced onion and a touch of olive oil.

- **Chill out.** Enjoy vegetarian bean chili with a dollop of low-fat or veggie sour cream or just add kidney beans to your favorite chili recipe.

- **Layer it up.** Layer vegetarian bean chili and rice, or chili and soy cheese with polenta to make an inside-out taco or polenta lasagna.

- **Pair them with whole grains.** Mix peas, pinto beans, garbanzo beans or kidney beans with corn, almond slivers and whole-wheat couscous; enjoy red beans with brown rice; or serve black beans with quinoa.

How to Pass on the Gas

While some can eat beans without suffering any ill effects, others get gas. That's because fiber goes right into their large intestine, where it's broken down and fermented by bacteria in intestinal flora, and this leads to the formation of carbon dioxide and other gases. Drinking water throughout the day can help fiber pass through your body, but eating beans in small amounts ($^1/_4$ cup counts as 1 Beans/Peas serving in the Vitality Diet) can also help. Beano can also help minimize gas and some of the gastrointestinal woes associated with eating beans.

SOYBEANS

In a review article published in *American Family Physician* in 2009, Aaron J. Michelfelder notes that populations with diets high in soy protein and low in animal protein have lower risks of prostate cancer and breast cancer than other populations. Although they have been consumed in China for more than a thousand years, soybeans and soy foods (including soy milk, tempeh and tofu) have yet to become dietary staples in the United States. But they have become more mainstream in recent years, thanks in part to the FDA's approval in 1999 of a health claim on food labels about the cholesterol-lowering effects of soy protein. Food manufacturers have responded to emerging research illustrating heart health, bone health, blood sugar and other benefits attributed to soy protein by providing options ranging from soy protein bars to veggie burgers to soy chips in order to please those who may not be sweet on whole soybeans and soy foods. But while soybeans, like other legumes, aren't likely to become dietary staples in the United States anytime soon, there's good reason to fit them—particularly in their traditional forms—into your Vitality Diet.

Unlike most plant foods, soybeans are a rich source of "high-quality" protein and supply all the amino acids the body needs to perform vital functions. (Some amino acids must be derived from the diet because they cannot be made in the body.) Soybeans also contain complex carbohydrates, which provide energy, as well as a healthy dose of both soluble and insoluble fiber. In addition they provide some essential dietary fats (those we need to obtain from the diet)—about half from the omega-6 fatty acid linoleic acid, a small amount of the omega-3 fatty acid ALA and some monounsaturated fatty acids. Soybeans have little saturated fat and no cholesterol.

Vital Stats: Soybeans and Soyfoods

Below you'll find the vital stats for various soyfoods:

Food	Calories	Protein (g)	Total Fat (g)	Carbohydrate (g)	Fiber (g)	Sugars (g)	Sodium (mg)	Daily Values*
Edamame (¼ cup)	47	4.2	2	3.9	2	<1	2	Excellent source of folate; Good source of manganese and vitamin K
Miso (fermented soybean paste) (1 Tbsp)	34	2	1	4.5	<1	1.1	634	N/A[1]
Soybeans, mature, boiled (¼ cup)	74	7.2	3.9	4.3	2.6	1.3	0	Good source of manganese, iron and phosphorus
Soy milk, original and vanilla (1 cup)	104	6.3	3.6	12	<1	8.9	114	Excellent source of vitamin B_{12}, calcium, riboflavin, vitamin D and copper; Good source of phosphorus

Food	Calories	Protein (g)	Total Fat (g)	Carbohydrate (g)	Fiber (g)	Sugars (g)	Sodium (mg)	Daily Values*
Soy milk, plain fortified (1 cup)	68	6	<1	10.1	<1	8.9	139	Excellent source of calcium, vitamin D and phosphorus; Good source of copper and vitamin A
Soy nuts, roasted, unsalted (2 Tbsp)	102	7.6	5.5	7.2	3.8	0	1	Excellent source of manganese; Good source of folate
Tempeh (1 ounce)	55	5.1	3.2	2.6	0	0	4	Good source of manganese
Tofu (¼ cup)	44	5.2	2.6	1.1	<1	<1	8	Good source of manganese and calcium

*An excellent source means the food contains > 20% of the Daily Value of a nutrient; a good source means the food contains 10-19% of a nutrient.

Source: U.S. Department of Agriculture, Agricultural Research Service. 2012. USDA National Nutrient Database for Standard Reference, Release 25. Nutrient Data Laboratory Home Page, www.ars.usda.gov/ba/bhnrc/ndi.

Sweet green soybeans (edamame) are an excellent source of folate and a good source of manganese and vitamin K, and mature soybeans provide a good amount of manganese and iron.

BENEFITS BEYOND THE LABEL

Soybeans are also important sources of isoflavones, which are phytoestrogens. Isoflavones have been studied for their role in protecting heart health and bone health and helping women manage those inconvenient menopausal hot flashes. A recent review published in *Menopause* in 2011 found soy-based isoflavones to be modestly effective in relieving menopausal symptoms. It also noted that the bone-protective effects of isoflavones have not yet been proven, and that the role of soy in cardiovascular health is still evolving. In a review in *Climacteric* in 2011, researchers analyzed several studies and found that most suggested a protective role for isoflavones in bone health. In a review that appeared in *Therapeutic Advances in Musculoskeletal Disease* in 2011, researchers concluded that soy foods are associated with improved bone health and that consuming them regularly as part of a diet rich in whole plant foods would likely optimize bone health.

Isoflavones found in soy foods were also shown to have antiaging properties—at least in mice—in a study published in the *Journal of the American College of Nutrition* in 2004. Researchers determined that isoflavones helped reduce the breakdown of collagen—a protein that is vital to keeping skin looking smooth, supple and youthful—caused by UV radiation. According to a 2008 article in *Obesity Reviews,* other studies have also shown that soy foods are as beneficial as other protein sources when it comes to weight loss.

Shopping for Soy

To derive the full benefits of soy (including soy protein and isoflavones), you may want to choose whole soy foods over other options, at least most of the time. According to the United Soybean Board, soy protein levels can be very small in processed soy foods, since they're added for functional purposes rather than nutritional ones. Registered dietitian Meredith Sobel, MS, RD, CDN, prefers whole soy foods, traditionally consumed in China and Japan, rather than processed soy foods. To help clients consume more soy, Sobel suggests combining some soy sauce, peanut butter (or almond butter) with a little milk or soy milk to make a sauce and serving the sauce on tofu, tempeh or plain soybeans, which can be paired with green vegetables. She also recommends eating edamame with either a green salad garnished with feta cheese and a splash of lemon, or with brown rice and broccoli, both quick and easy meals.

LEAN BEEF

Despite the bad rap red meat tends to get, lean beef has several virtues that earn it a supporting role in your Vitality Diet. The American Heart Association recommends lean beef, along with lean pork or lamb, poultry and fish, as a daily option, and lean beef is also included as a protein option in current Dietary Guidelines for Americans. The Adult Treatment Panel III Guidelines of the National Cholesterol Education Program (NCEP) agree that lean beef can be part of a heart-healthy diet and that there's no need to dramatically reduce or cut consumption. And while the American Institute for Cancer Research (AICR) recommends avoiding processed meats, they say it's okay to include red meat—including lean beef, lamb and pork—in your weekly diet, but to limit it to no more than eighteen ounces cooked each week to reduce cancer risk.

When you take a close look at the nutritional profile of lean beef, you'll see that top sirloin and other popular cuts provide fewer calories, less total fat and saturated fat, less cholesterol, and more Vital Nutrients than you might have imagined. Lean beef is an excellent source of high-quality protein. A three-ounce portion (the size of a small palm) of the ever-popular cut top sirloin contains 140 calories and only four grams of total fat. About two thirds of the fat is heart-healthy monounsaturated fat and polyunsaturated fat, and only one-third is saturated fat—the kind we limit because of its link with heart disease. Top sirloin is also an excellent source of selenium, niacin, zinc, vitamin B_6, vitamin B_{12} and phosphorus and has smaller amounts of several other nutrients.

BEEF BENEFITS

Recent studies suggest that lean beef can be a vital part of a nutritious, high-quality diet. In a study published in *Meat Science* in 2012, consuming lean beef was shown to contribute significant amounts of protein, vitamin B_{12}, zinc, iron, niacin, vitamin B_6, phosphorus and potassium to the diets of American adults. Consuming lean beef has also been shown to benefit blood cholesterol (surprise, surprise!). The Beef in an Optimal Lean Diet (BOLD) study, published in the *American Journal of Clinical Nutrition* in 2012, found that consuming lean beef (about 4 to 5.4 ounces before cooking) daily as part of a heart-healthy diet was just as effective at lowering total cholesterol and LDL (bad) cholesterol as the well-known Dietary Approaches to Stop Hypertension (DASH) diet in adults who had moderately elevated cholesterol levels. A few studies have also illustrated how eating beef preserves muscle. A study published in the *Journal of Nutrition, Health & Aging* in 2012 found a positive association between beef consumption and muscle mass measured by mid-arm muscle area. Total protein intake was also positively correlated with nutrition status, calf circumference and BMI in older adults.

In another study, this one published in the *Journal of the American Dietetic Association* in 2009, researchers found that a single moderate (4½ ounces) serving of 90 percent lean beef increased muscle protein synthesis by approximately 50 percent in both young and older subjects. No further increase in muscle protein synthesis was seen in the subjects after ingesting the larger serving (12 ounces) of beef. And a study published in the *British*

Journal of Nutrition showed that consuming adequate protein from lean beef and other foods enhanced the muscle-preserving benefits of muscle-strengthening or resistance exercise in more than twenty-four hundred adults aged fifty and older. Furthermore, a study published in the *American Journal of Clinical Nutrition* in 2007 found that consuming four ounces of lean beef acutely stimulated muscle protein synthesis by 50 percent in both young and elderly volunteers. The researchers concluded that including high-quality protein foods, such as lean beef, in each meal is a practical dietary strategy to stimulate muscle growth, optimize muscle strength and metabolism, and ultimately improve overall health.

If you enjoy beef, eat it! Just try to aim as often as possible for the leanest cuts (see Where's the (Lean) Beef?), and choose those instead of processed meats most (if not all) of the time to maximize benefits and minimize potential perils associated with high red meat intake. Although the Vitality Diet has no hard and fast rule for lean beef intake, a good rule of thumb is to have up to six ounces weekly if you choose to have it. That gives you your protein fix but also leaves room for other vital protein foods, like eggs, poultry, beans and peas, fish, and nuts and seeds. And when you cook lean beef, you can minimize your exposure to potentially dangerous, cancer-causing chemicals such as heterocyclic amines (HCAs) and polycyclic aromatic hydrocarbons (PAHs), which can form when meats, fish and poultry are cooked at high temperatures, by using smaller pieces, trimming fat, using certain herbs (such as rosemary) and/or marinades, precooking the beef in a microwave, cooking it at a lower temperature and for less time, and flipping it often.

Where's the (Lean) Beef?

According to the USDA, three ounces cooked lean beef is "lean" if it has < 10 grams of fat, < 4.5 grams of saturated fat, and < 95 milligrams of cholesterol and is "extra lean" if it provides < 5 grams of fat, < 2 grams of saturated fat, and < 95 milligrams of cholesterol.
Below you'll find the cuts that qualify as "lean" or "extra lean" beef:

Cut (3 ounces, cooked*)	Total Fat (grams)	Saturated Fat (grams)
Beef eye round roast and steak**	4	1.4
Beef top round roast	4.3	1.5
Beef top round steak	4.6	1.6

Cut (3 ounces, cooked*)	Total Fat (grams)	Saturated Fat (grams)
Beef bottom round roast	4.9	1.7
Beef top sirloin steak	5	1.9
Beef chuck shoulder steak	5	2.1
Beef round steak/cubed steak	5.3	1.9
Beef round tip roast and steak	5.3	1.9
Beef shank cross cuts	5.4	1.9
Beef bottom round (western griller) steak	6	2.2
Beef top loin (strip) steak	6	2.3
Beef flank steak	6.3	2.6
Beef bottom round steak	6.6	2.3
Beef tenderloin roast and steak	6.7	2.5
Beef brisket, flat half	6.8	2.7
93% lean ground beef patty	6.8	2.9
Beef tri-tip roast and steak	7.1	2.6
Beef T-bone steak	7.4	2.6
Beef boneless top blade steak	7.9	3.2

*Visible fat removed.

**Cuts combined for illustration purposes.

Source: US Department of Agriculture, Agricultural Research Service, 2012. USDA Nutrient Database for Standard Reference, Release 25. Nutrient Data Laboratory. Homepage www.ars.usda.gov/ba/bhnrc/ndl.

Information courtesy of The Beef Checkoff.

Do 'Em or Ditch 'Em?

Processed Meats

A review article published in *Circulation* in 2010 evaluated twenty studies that included more than 1.2 million subjects to determine the association between total meat intake, unprocessed red meat

continued on page 82

intake, and processed meat intake and the risk of coronary heart disease and diabetes. While no association was found between a daily intake of 3.5 ounces of unprocessed red meat and the incidence of coronary heart disease and diabetes, each daily serving of processed meat (for example, one hot dog or 50 g [~1.8 oz] of bacon or salami) was associated with a 42 percent higher coronary heart disease risk and a 19 percent higher diabetes risk. According to the World Cancer Research Fund/American Institute for Cancer Research's Continuous Update Project (CUP), a review of more than one thousand studies on colorectal cancer found convincing evidence that both red and processed meat increase colorectal cancer risk. According to Karen Collins, MS, RD, CDN, nutrition advisor for the American Institute for Cancer Research (AICR), "Processed meat—meat that is smoked, salted, cured or with added preservatives like nitrites—may increase colorectal cancer risk, because compounds used as preservatives may change into cancer-causing compounds in the body. Excess amounts of unprocessed red meat may also increase cancer risk because of high-heat cooking methods that create cancer-causing compounds or because they're high in heme iron, which may promote the formation of certain carcinogens within the gut and generate free radicals." While the AICR urges Americans to limit red meat, as discussed on page 78, it also recommends avoiding processed meats, such as ham, bacon, pastrami, salami, hot dogs and sausages. The bottom line? Ditch 'em if you can live without them, but do 'em if you must—but only once in a while (have a hot dog at a baseball game or enjoy half of a salami sandwich when you're visiting your favorite New York City deli).

Chicken, Turkey and the "Other" White Meats

Not only do poultry (including chicken and turkey) and pork loin provide high-quality protein, but they're also excellent sources of selenium, niacin and vitamin B_6, and good sources of phosphorus. Pork loin is also an excellent source of thiamine and a good source of zinc and riboflavin. Choose skinless, lower-fat poultry—breast meat, for example—and opt for those brands prepared with less sodium. If you consume cold cuts, opt for brands without added nitrates or nitrites, potentially cancer-causing chemicals that naturally occur in water and food (including vegetables) and are added to many processed meats.

Protein

Aim for about six servings of protein a day (see Chapter 12). To meet that goal, choose at least two ½-ounce servings of nuts, nut butters and seeds* daily; 1½ cups of beans/peas weekly; and eight to twelve ounces of fish/shellfish weekly. Emphasize protein-rich foods during the day to stay awake and alert. See Chapter 12 for a list of recommended protein sources and be sure to incorporate some protein into each meal or snack.

*Nuts, nut butters and seeds also count as sources of Healthy Fats (see Chapters 4 and 12).

DON'T WORRY, B-HAPPY

B vitamins—and the foods that contain them—are key components of the Vitality Diet for so many reasons. I like to call B vitamins the body's Energizer Bunnies because they help turn the food we eat into usable energy. But they are also involved in a wide variety of body functions that keep your skin smooth, your hair healthy, your brain nourished and your mood on an even keel. We need to consume these nutrients daily since most aren't stored in the body. But don't worry—the Vitality Diet is packed with plenty of B-rich foods to make it a breeze to get your Bs.

Although foods rich in B vitamins are plentiful—these include enriched and fortified grains and lean beef, as well as salmon and soybeans—many women are at risk of falling short on them. For example, you may be at risk for inadequate vitamin B_{12} intake if you don't consume any or enough grains or if you regularly drink too much alcohol. Also, as you grow older, your body has more difficulty absorbing vitamin B_{12} from food. And there's evidence that not getting enough of certain B vitamins can cause a litany of vitality-sapping troubles that take their toll on your hair, skin, vision, appetite, mood and even your ability to sleep. Not getting enough of your Bs also can contribute to the development of cardio-vascular disease and even Alzheimer's disease, but why play "wait and see" when there are steps you can take today to take charge of your health and well-being?

Studies suggest that not getting enough of vital B vitamins—especially vitamin B_6, folate and vitamin B_{12}—can sap your vitality by contributing to depression, exacerbating stress and burdening your brain.

B VITAMINS AND DEPRESSION

Several studies have posited a connection between B vitamins and depression. A study published in *Psychotherapy and Psychosomatics* in 2004 found that low plasma levels of pyridoxal phosphate (PLP)—a measure of vitamin B_6 in the body—was associated with symptoms of depression. A deficiency of vitamin B_{12} and, to a lesser extent, a folate deficiency were also found to be related to depressive disorders in a study of more than 3,800 elderly people that appeared in the *American Journal of Psychiatry* in 2002. The study also found an association between high levels of the amino acid homocysteine and depression. B vitamins, especially vitamin B_{12}, folate and vitamin B_6, play central roles in regulating homocysteine levels in the blood, and some studies suggest that high levels of homocysteine contribute significantly to depression risk.

B VITAMINS AND YOUR PSYCHE

Although the data on psychological stress and B vitamin intake is scarce, a few studies suggest that lower levels of B vitamins (particularly folate, vitamin B_{12} and vitamin B_6) may be key contributors to future stress. In a 2009 study published in *Public Health Nutrition,* researchers determined that a low dietary intake of vitamin B_{12} in middle-aged women was associated with higher psychological distress at that age. A study in the *Journal of the American Dietetic Association* in 2010 found that among Vietnamese women, those with the most psychological distress had a lower consumption of nutrients, including thiamine, riboflavin and folate, compared to women with the lowest stress scores. Given that vitamin B_6 is crucial for the creation of serotonin and other mood-regulating neurotransmitters, inadequate levels of the vitamin likely reduce serotonin levels in the brain, which can contribute to psychological distress.

B VITAMINS AND YOUR BRAIN

Deficiencies of some B vitamins, especially folate, vitamin B_{12} and vitamin B_6, have been linked with impaired cognition and increased levels of homocysteine, which not only harms the heart but also may contribute to the risk of Alzheimer's disease earlier in life. A 2013 study published in *Psychosomatic Medicine* found that low vitamin B_{12} status was associated with cognitive deficit among more than nineteen hundred adults aged seventy-one to seventy-four. And a study that appeared in *Neurology* in 2011 concluded that vitamin B_{12} status was a risk factor for changes in the brain that could contribute to cognitive impairment.

Fortunately, the news about B vitamins isn't all bleak. A few studies suggest that help may actually "B" on the way when it comes to beating the blues, fighting PMS and keeping your brain sharp. Here are just a few findings:

- In a study published in 2010 in the *American Journal of Clinical Nutrition*, researchers investigated whether dietary intakes of vitamins B_6, folate or vitamin B_{12} predicted symptoms of depression in more than thirty-five hundred adults aged sixty-five and older. They found that over seven years, higher intakes of vitamin B_6 and vitamin B_{12} from food and supplements combined were associated with a lower likelihood of depression.

- In a 2011 study that appeared in the *American Journal of Clinical Nutrition*, researchers evaluated whether the intake of B vitamins from food sources or supplements was associated with the initial development of PMS—that uncomfortable premenstrual cluster of physical and psychological symptoms (can you say bloat and the blues?), which is estimated to affect about 15 percent of women in their reproductive years. Researchers found that in a sample of almost 117,000 women who were followed for ten years, those with the highest intakes of riboflavin from foods were 35 percent less likely to develop PMS than those who had the lowest intakes. Similarly, women who had the highest intakes of thiamine were 25 percent less likely to develop PMS than those with the lowest intakes. Researchers suggested these intake levels could be achieved by consuming two to three daily servings of thiamine-rich foods (such as fortified cereals, legumes, nuts, and pork or other red meats) and six to seven daily servings of riboflavin-rich foods (such as cow's milk, soy milk, spinach or red meats).

- Having high plasma levels of thiamine, riboflavin, vitamin B_6, folate and vitamin B_{12} was shown to confer brain-boosting benefits in elderly men and women, according to a study published in *Neurology* in 2012.

Vitality Check ✓

Why You Might Need More Bs

If you follow a vegetarian or vegan diet that allows little or no animal foods, or if you're at risk for being or are deficient in vitamin B_{12} (individuals aged fifty and older have a reduced ability to absorb the nutrient from food), you probably won't be able to meet all your B needs through diet alone. If that's the case, see your doctor (and a registered dietitian) to discuss supplementation before you add any vitamin or mineral supplement to your daily repertoire. (See Appendix C for guidelines on your daily nutrient needs.)

ALL ABOUT THE Bs

In the pages that follow, you'll learn more about the vital B vitamins—thiamine, riboflavin, niacin, pantothenic acid, biotin, vitamin B_6, folate and vitamin B_{12}—what they do and where you'll find them so that you can reap their many age-defying and mood-boosting benefits.

THIAMINE

Also known as vitamin B_1, thiamine helps convert carbohydrates in food into energy. It also helps enzymes maintain functions of the muscles, nerves and the heart. In addition, thiamine is needed for healthy skin and nails. Although a thiamine deficiency is rare, alcoholics are at risk. Deficiency symptoms may include fatigue, muscle weakness and nerve damage.

Thiamin-Rich Foods

Here you'll find food sources that provide at least 10 percent of the Daily Value* (1.5 milligrams) of thiamine. (Any mention of brand-name items should not be construed as an implied endorsement.)

Food	Protein	Thiamin (mg)	Daily Value (%)**
Raisin bran cereal	1 cup	1.54	103
General Mills Wheaties	1 cup	0.84	56
Rice, white, long-grain, parboiled, enriched, dried	½ cup	0.56	37
Pork chop, bone in, lean, cooked	3 ounces	0.48	32
Oats, instant, fortified, plain, prepared with water	1 packet	0.46	31
Spaghetti, cooked, without added salt	1 cup	0.38	26
Kellogg's Frosted Mini-Wheats, Bite Size or Little Bites	1 cup	0.38	25
Kaiser roll	1 roll	0.27	18
Salmon, sockeye, cooked	4 ounces	0.24	16
Soybeans, green, boiled, drained, without salt	½ cup	0.23	16
Peas, green, frozen, boiled without salt	½ cup	0.23	15
Cowpeas (black-eyed peas), immature seeds, frozen, cooked without salt	½ cup	0.22	15
Black beans, mature seeds, cooked without salt	½ cup	0.22	14
Navy beans, mature seeds, cooked without salt	½ cup	0.22	14
Okra, cooked without salt	1 cup	0.21	14
Macadamia nuts, dry roasted, unsalted	1 ounce	0.20	13
Pistachio nuts, dry roasted, unsalted	1 ounce	0.20	13
Pecans	1 ounce	0.19	13
Split peas, mature seeds, cooked without salt	½ cup	0.19	12
Brazil nuts, dried, unblanched	1 ounce	0.18	12
Hazelnuts (filberts)	1 ounce	0.18	12
Lentils, mature seeds, cooked without salt	½ cup	0.17	11

Food	Protein	Thiamin (mg)	Daily Value (%)**
Pinto beans, mature seeds, cooked without salt	½ cup	0.17	11
Lima beans, mature seeds, cooked without salt	½ cup	0.15	10

*Foods that provide 10 to 19 percent of the Daily Value of a nutrient are good sources. Foods that provide at least 20 percent of the Daily Value of a nutrient are excellent sources.

**Daily Value percentages are rounded to the nearest whole number.

Source: U.S. Department of Agriculture, Agricultural Research Service. 2012. USDA National Nutrient Database for Standard Reference, Release 25. Nutrient Data Laboratory Home Page, www.ars.usda.gov/nutrientdata.

RIBOFLAVIN

This B vitamin, also known as vitamin B_2, helps turn carbohydrates into energy. It also helps in the formation of red blood cells, which carry oxygen throughout the body and are involved in several important chemical reactions in the body. In addition, riboflavin supports healthy skin and helps maintain vision. Symptoms of a deficiency can include anemia, skin disorders, sores in your mouth or on your lips, tired eyes or sensitivity to light.

Riboflavin-Rich Foods

Here you'll find food sources that provide at least 10 percent of the Daily Value* (1.7 milligrams) of riboflavin. (Any mention of brand-name items should not be construed as an implied endorsement.)

Food	Portion	Riboflavin (mg)	Daily Value (%)**
General Mills Total Whole Grain	1 cup	2.27	134
Raisin bran cereal	1 cup	1.76	104
General Mills Wheaties	1 cup	0.93	55
Yogurt, plain, low-fat or nonfat	1 cup	0.53	31
Milk, low-fat or nonfat	1 cup	0.45	26
Kellogg's Frosted Mini-Wheats, Bite Size or Little Bites	1 cup	0.43	25

continued on page 90

Food	Portion	Riboflavin (mg)	Daily Value (%)**
Oats, instant, fortified, plain, prepared with water	1 packet	0.38	22
Spinach, frozen, chopped or whole leaf, cooked without salt	1 cup	0.33	20
Almonds	1 ounce	0.29	17
Egg, whole, hard-boiled or scrambled	1 large	0.26	16
Sardines, Atlantic, canned, drained	4 ounces	0.26	15
Mushrooms, shiitake, cooked without salt	1 cup	0.25	15
Puffed wheat or puffed rice cereal	1 cup	0.25	15
Soybeans, mature, boiled without salt	½ cup	0.25	14
Feta cheese	1 ounce	0.24	14
Collards, cooked without salt	1 cup	0.20	12
Broccoli, cooked without salt	1 cup	0.19	11
Cottage cheese, low-fat or nonfat	½ cup	0.19	11
Spaghetti or macaroni, cooked without salt	1 cup	0.19	11
Prune juice, canned	1 cup	0.18	11
Okra, frozen, cooked without salt	1 cup	0.18	10
Brussels sprouts, frozen, cooked without salt	1 cup	0.18	10

*Foods that provide 10 to 19 percent of the Daily Value of a nutrient are good sources. Foods that provide at least 20 percent of the Daily Value of a nutrient are excellent sources.

**Daily Value percentages are rounded to the nearest whole number.

Source: U.S. Department of Agriculture, Agricultural Research Service. 2012. USDA National Nutrient Database for Standard Reference, Release 25. Nutrient Data Laboratory Home Page, www.ars.usda.gov/nutrientdata.

NIACIN

Also called vitamin B_3, niacin, like other B vitamins, helps turn the food we eat into energy. It works with enzymes in several important chemical reactions. Niacin also supports skin health and aids digestion and nerve function. Although a deficiency of this vitamin is uncommon, symptoms may include scaly skin, digestive problems, such as diarrhea and vomiting, headache, fatigue, depression and poor memory. Niacin deficiency may also contribute to a depletion of tryptophan, needed to create serotonin.

Niacin-Rich Foods

Here you'll find food sources that provide at least 10 percent of the Daily Value* (20 milligrams) of niacin. (Any mention of brand-name items should not be construed as an implied endorsement.)

Food	Portion	Niacin (mg)	Daily Value (%)**
General Mills Total Whole Grain	1 cup	26.67	133
Raisin bran cereal	1 cup	20.75	104
Tuna, light, canned in water, drained	4 ounces	15.05	75
Salmon, sockeye, cooked	4 ounces	10.99	55
Halibut, Atlantic or Pacific, cooked over dry heat	4 ounces	8.97	45
Pork loin, bone-in, lean, cooked	3 ounces	8.50	43
Rainbow trout, farmed, cooked	4 ounces	7.53	38
Pink salmon, canned	4 ounces	7.40	37
Pork chop, lean, broiled	3 ounces	7.20	36
Top sirloin, steak, lean, cooked	3 ounces	7.16	36
Ground turkey, cooked	1 patty (about 3 ounces)	7.15	36
Mushrooms, white, cooked without salt	1 cup	6.96	35
Tuna, white, canned in water, drained	4 ounces	6.57	33
Sardines, Atlantic, canned in oil, drained	4 ounces	5.95	30
Lamb, loin, lean, cooked	3 ounces	5.82	29
Oats, instant, fortified, plain, prepared with water	1 cup	5.35	27
Bottom round, steak, lean, cooked	3 ounces	5.24	26
Spaghetti (or marinara) sauce	½ cup	4.89	25
Peanuts, dry-roasted without salt	1 ounce	3.83	19

continued on page 92

Food	Portion	Niacin (mg)	Daily Value (%)**
Crab, blue, cooked	4 ounces	3.11	16
Potato, baked without salt	1 potato	2.85	14
Shredded wheat cereal	2 biscuits	2.41	12
Peanut butter, chunky style, with salt	1 tablespoon	2.19	11
Mushrooms, shiitake, cooked without salt	1 cup	2.18	11
Sweet potatoes, baked in skin without salt	1 potato	2.17	11
Peanut butter, smooth style, with salt	1 tablespoon	2.14	10
White rice, long-grain, enriched, cooked	½ cup	2.02	10
Prune juice, canned	1 cup	2.01	10

*Foods that provide 10 to 19 percent of the Daily Value of a nutrient are good sources. Foods that provide at least 20 percent of the Daily Value of a nutrient are excellent sources.

**Daily Value percentages are rounded to the nearest whole number.

Source: U.S. Department of Agriculture, Agricultural Research Service. 2012. USDA National Nutrient Database for Standard Reference, Release 25. Nutrient Data Laboratory Home Page, www.ars.usda.gov/nutrientdata.

PANTOTHENIC ACID

Pantothenic acid, sometimes called vitamin B_5, creates energy from carbohydrates, fat and protein. It also helps produce hormones (messengers that carry information from place to place around the body), essential fats (such as phospholipids, which are key components of cell membranes) and cholesterol. Although a deficiency of this vitamin is uncommon, symptoms can include fatigue, nausea, abdominal cramps, sleep troubles or numbness in the extremities.

Pantothenic Acid–Rich Foods

Here you'll find food sources that provide at least 10 percent of the Daily Value* (10 milligrams) of pantothenic acid. (Any mention of brand-name items should not be construed as an implied endorsement.)

Food	Portion	Pantothenic Acid (mg)	Daily Value (%)**
General Mills Total Whole Grain	1 cup	13.33	133
Raisin bran cereal	1 cup	10.37	104
Mushrooms, shiitake, cooked without salt	1 cup	5.21	52
Mushrooms, white, cooked	1 cup	3.37	34
Rainbow trout, farmed, cooked over dry heat	4 ounces	2.26	23
Lobster, Northern, cooked	4 ounces	1.89	19
Salmon, sockeye, cooked over dry heat	4 ounces	1.55	16
Yogurt, nonfat	1 cup	1.45	15
Yogurt, plain, low-fat	1 cup	1.34	13
Pork loin, lean, bone-in, cooked	3 ounces	1.33	13
Sweet potato, canned	1 cup	1.33	13
Sweet potatoes, baked in skin	1 potato	1.29	13
Mushrooms, canned, drained	1 cup	1.27	13
Sunflower seeds, dry-roasted, with salt added	2 tablespoons	1.13	11
Blue crab, canned	4 ounces	1.10	11

*Foods that provide 10 to 19 percent of the Daily Value of a nutrient are good sources. Foods that provide at least 20 percent of the Daily Value of a nutrient are excellent sources.

**Daily Value percentages are rounded to the nearest whole number.

Source: U.S. Department of Agriculture, Agricultural Research Service. 2012. USDA National Nutrient Database for Standard Reference, Release 25. Nutrient Data Laboratory Home Page, www.ars.usda.gov/nutrientdata.

BIOTIN

Although most biotin is derived from the diet, your body makes some of it. This B vitamin works with several enzymes to turn carbohydrates into usable energy, produce fatty acids and create or metabolize amino acids. It also supports the functions of DNA. Signs of a biotin deficiency may include hair loss, scaly skin, depression, loss of appetite and lethargy. Those who eat a lot of raw egg whites—something I discourage to reduce the risk of contamination from salmonella—may be at risk for a biotin deficiency, since avidin, a protein found in raw egg whites, prevents biotin absorption. (Cooking eggs, however, inactivates avidin.)

Although the amounts of biotin in food are largely unknown, research suggests that meat, fish, poultry, eggs, dairy and some vegetables are rich sources.

VITAMIN B$_6$

Also known as pyroxidine, vitamin B$_6$ has many roles in your body. It works with enzymes that perform several chemical reactions. It helps create glucose from glycogen (stored glucose). It is instrumental in the formation of heme, the iron-containing part of hemoglobin, which is found in red blood cells, through which oxygen is delivered throughout the body. Vitamin B$_6$ is also involved in neurotransmitter syntheses: it helps turn tryptophan into serotonin and supports other enzymes in the creation of other neurotransmitters, including dopamine, norepinephrine and GABA. It may also aid in the conversion of the omega-3 fatty acid ALA into DHA, a more potent omega-3 fatty acid. A deficiency of vitamin B$_6$, though uncommon, can contribute to irritability, depression, confusion, and inflammation in and around the mouth.

Vitamin B$_6$–Rich Foods

Here you'll find food sources that provide at least 10 percent of the Daily Value* (2 milligrams) of vitamin B$_6$. (Any mention of brand-name items should not be construed as an implied endorsement.)

Food	Portion	Vitamin B$_6$ (mg)	Daily Value (%)**
General Mills Total Whole Grain	1 cup	2.67	134
Raisin bran cereal	1 cup	2.07	104
Tuna, yellowfin, cooked	4 ounces	1.18	59

Food	Portion	Vitamin B$_6$ (mg)	Daily Value (%)**
General Mills Wheaties	1 cup	1.11	56
Salmon, sockeye, cooked	4 ounces	0.79	39
Halibut, Atlantic or Pacific, cooked	4 ounces	0.72	36
Potatoes, baked	1 potato	0.63	31
Pork chop, lean, cooked	3 ounces	0.60	30
Chickpeas (garbanzo beans), mature seeds, canned, solids and liquids	½ cup	0.57	29
Bananas, raw	1 cup	0.55	28
Top sirloin, lean, cooked	3 ounces	0.54	27
Kellogg's Frosted Mini-Wheats	1 cup	0.52	26
Oats, instant, fortified, plain, prepared with water	1 packet	0.51	26
Turkey, light meat, cooked	3 ounces	0.45	23
Brussels sprouts, frozen, cooked	1 cup	0.45	22
Rainbow trout, farmed, cooked	4 ounces	0.44	22
Spinach, cooked	1 cup	0.44	22
Peppers, sweet, red, raw	1 cup	0.43	22
Sweet potatoes, baked	1 cup	0.42	21
Potatoes, boiled	1 potato	0.41	21
Beef, bottom round, lean, cooked	3 ounces	0.39	20
Haddock, cooked over dry heat	4 ounces	0.37	19
Plaintains, cooked	1 cup	0.37	19
Beef, round, eye of round, lean, cooked	3 ounces	0.34	17
Squash, winter, all varieties, cooked	1 cup	0.33	17
Pistachio nuts, dry-roasted, with salt added	1 ounce	0.32	16

continued on page 96

Food	Portion	Vitamin B_6 (mg)	Daily Value (%)**
Broccoli, cooked	1 cup	0.31	16
Soybeans, mature, boiled	½ cup	0.20	10

*Foods that provide 10 to 19 percent of the Daily Value of a nutrient are good sources. Foods that provide at least 20 percent of the Daily Value of a nutrient are excellent sources.

**Daily Value percentages are rounded to the nearest whole number.

Source: U.S. Department of Agriculture, Agricultural Research Service. 2012. USDA National Nutrient Database for Standard Reference, Release 25. Nutrient Data Laboratory Home Page, www.ars.usda.gov/nutrientdata.

FOLATE

In addition to its key role in preventing neural tube defects in fetuses during early pregnancy, folate works with vitamin B_{12} and vitamin C to help your body use and produce new proteins. It also facilitates the formation of red blood cells, helps cells grow and divide, and helps lower homocysteine levels, which may protect both your heart and your brain. Folate also plays an integral role in the creation of neurotransmitters, including serotonin, epinephrine and dopamine. A folate deficiency can contribute to birth defects and anemia, with symptoms including weakness, fatigue, depression, irritability, forgetfulness and disturbed sleep. A lack of folate can also impair DNA synthesis and contribute to cardiovascular disease and Alzheimer's disease. And a folate deficiency can wreak havoc with your mood because of altered neurotransmitter synthesis. Alcoholics are at risk for a folate deficiency, as are those who don't consume any or enough folate-rich foods or the more highly absorbed folic acid in fortified foods or supplements.

Folate-Rich Foods

Here you'll find food sources that provide at least 10 percent of the Daily Value* (400 micrograms) of folate. (Any mention of brand-name items should not be construed as an implied endorsement.)

Food	Portion	Folate (mcg)	Daily Value (%)**
Okra, cooked	1 cup	184	46

Food	Portion	Folate (mcg)	Daily Value (%)**
Lentils, mature seeds, cooked	1/2 cup	179	45
Collard greens, cooked	1 cup	177	44
Turnip greens, cooked	1 cup	170	43
Broccoli, cooked	1 cup	168	42
Kellogg's Frosted Mini-Wheats	1 cup	167	42
Spaghetti, enriched, cooked	1 cup	167	42
Artichokes, globe or French, cooked	1 cup	150	38
Pinto beans, mature seeds, cooked	1/2 cup	147	37
Beets, cooked	1 cup	136	34
Black beans, mature seeds, cooked	1/2 cup	128	32
Navy beans, mature seeds, cooked	1/2 cup	128	32
Oats, instant, fortified, plain, prepared with water	1 cup	126	32
Red kidney beans, mature seeds, cooked	1/2 cup	115	29
Cowpeas (black-eyed peas), immature seeds, cooked	1/2 cup	105	26
Soybeans, green, cooked	1/2 cup	100	25
Great Northern beans, mature seeds, cooked	1/2 cup	91	23
White beans, mature seeds, cooked	1/2 cup	85	21
Split peas, mature seeds, cooked, boiled	1/2 cup	64	16
Cowpeas (black-eyed peas), mature seeds, canned	1/2 cup	61	15
Lima beans, canned	1/2 cup	61	15

*Foods that provide 10 to 19 percent of the Daily Value of a nutrient are good sources. Foods that provide at least 20 percent of the Daily Value of a nutrient are excellent sources.

**Daily Value percentages are rounded to the nearest whole number.

Source: U.S. Department of Agriculture, Agricultural Research Service. 2012. USDA National Nutrient Database for Standard Reference, Release 25. Nutrient Data Laboratory Home Page, www.ars.usda.gov/nutrientdata.

VITAMIN B$_{12}$

Vitamin B$_{12}$ plays a vital role in helping the body grow and develop. Like other B vitamins, it helps the body make energy from food. It also plays a vital part in the production of red blood cells and supports nervous system function, especially by working with enzymes (and other B vitamins, including vitamin B$_6$ and folate) to make and maintain serotonin and other neurotransmitters. And vitamin B$_{12}$ helps regulate homocysteine levels.

Vitamin B$_{12}$–Rich Foods

Here you'll find food sources that provide at least 10 percent of the Daily Value* (6 micrograms) of vitamin B$_{12}$. (Any mention of brand-name items should not be construed as an implied endorsement.)

Food	Portion	Vitamin B$_{12}$ (mcg)	Daily Value (%)**
Tuna, yellowfin, cooked	4 ounces	2.66	44
Cod, Pacific, cooked	4 ounces	2.61	44
Tuna, light, canned in oil, drained	4 ounces	2.49	42
Beef, chuck, lean, cooked	3 ounces	2.10	35
Cheerios	1 cup	1.86	31
Lamb, lean, cooked	3 ounces	1.84	31
Lobster, Northern, cooked	4 ounces	1.63	27
Beef, round, bottom round, lean, cooked	3 ounces	1.61	27
Halibut, Atlantic or Pacific, cooked	4 ounces	1.44	24
Beef, top sirloin, lean, cooked	3 ounces	1.43	24
Yogurt, plain, nonfat	1 cup	1.38	23
Tuna, white, canned in water, drained solids	4 ounces	1.32	22
Yogurt, plain, low-fat	1 cup	1.27	21
Milk, nonfat	1 cup	1.23	21
Milk, low-fat	1 cup	1.15	19
Shrimp, canned	4 ounces	0.84	14

Food	Portion	Vitamin B$_{12}$ (mcg)	Daily Value (%)**
Chocolate milk, low-fat	1 cup	0.80	13
Cheese, mozzarella, whole milk or part skim	1 ounce	0.65	11

*Foods that provide 10 to 19 percent of the Daily Value of a nutrient are good sources. Foods that provide at least 20 percent of the Daily Value of a nutrient are excellent sources.

**Daily Value percentages are rounded to the nearest whole number.

Source: U.S. Department of Agriculture, Agricultural Research Service. 2012. USDA National Nutrient Database for Standard Reference, Release 25. Nutrient Data Laboratory Home Page, www.ars.usda.gov/nutrientdata.

Vital R$_x$

Don't Worry, B-Happy

Include oats or ready-to-eat whole-grain cereal as part of your starchy carb (see Chapter 3) allotment in your daily Vitality Diet. Oats provide an excellent dose of thiamine, riboflavin, niacin, vitamin B$_6$ and folate, and most whole-grain cereals are also good or excellent sources of these Vital Nutrients.

Consume fish and shellfish as part of your weekly protein intake (see Chapter 5). Tuna, salmon and halibut are rich in vitamin B$_6$, and tuna, halibut, cod, lobster and shrimp are rich in vitamin B$_{12}$.

If you limit or avoid animal foods and/or are aged fifty and older, discuss supplementation (especially of vitamin B$_{12}$) with a physician.

GET IN TUNE WITH YOUR PMS-C

No, I'm not talking about *that* PMS. I'm talking about four major minerals—potassium, magnesium, sodium and calcium. These micronutrients aren't needed in large amounts and they don't have the clout of energy-yielding carbohydrates, fat and protein. But potassium, magnesium, sodium and calcium play vital roles in the body, often working in tandem to do everything from supporting muscle and nerve function to regulating fluid balance. And, speaking of balance, consuming a diet that's rich in potassium, magnesium and calcium and moderate in sodium is a great way to keep your PMS-C levels in check, thereby supporting strong bones and muscles—including your heart—to keep you vibrant.

POTASSIUM

You may be surprised to learn that potassium helps virtually every body part function optimally. It supports muscle function and nerve function, helps your heart beat steadily and promotes fluid balance in the blood and in body tissues. Among its integral roles, potassium helps blunt the negative effects that too much sodium has on blood pressure. There's also evidence it can reduce the risk of stroke. Potassium also may play a role in preventing bone loss and reducing the risk of developing painful kidney stones.

Although low potassium levels can be a consequence of taking certain medications or diuretics, having certain medical conditions, or having too much licorice or herbal teas made with glycyrrhetinic acid, a poor dietary intake of vegetables, legumes and other potassium-rich foods can also contribute. And while a small drop in blood values for potassium may not cause any symptoms, a big drop can be life threatening and can lead to abnormal heart rhythms; constipation; fatigue; muscle weakness, spasms or damage; and even paralysis and cardiac arrest.

Vitality Check ✓

Do We Meet Our Potassium Needs?

Despite the fact that potassium is found in a wide variety of foods, including vegetables, fruits, legumes, fish and dairy products, national survey data from 2008 reveals that about 95 percent of Americans don't meet recommended intake levels, which is why the federal government considers potassium a "nutrient of concern." Given that potassium is critical to good health, it's important to increase your daily intake* of potassium-rich foods (see Potassium-Rich Foods on page 103) if you are one of the 95 percent. And since many potassium-rich foods—especially fresh fruits and vegetables and dried beans—are also low in sodium, choosing more of them kills two birds by also reducing sodium intake.

*If you have kidney disease or take any medications, consult with your doctor for guidance on potassium intake.

THE PERILS OF LOW-POTASSIUM, HIGH-SODIUM DIETS

Consuming too little potassium and at the same time having too much sodium can be a double curse when it comes to vitality. In a study published in the *Clinical Journal of the American Society of Nephrology* in 2012, researchers noted a significant increase in blood pressure with increases in the sodium/potassium ratio in thirty-three hundred middle-aged adults and concluded that too much dietary sodium and too little potassium may lead to hypertension. And in a study published in *Archives of Internal Medicine* in 2011, researchers followed more than twelve thousand adults for almost fifteen years and found that a higher sodium/potassium ratio based on typical dietary intake was associated with a 50 percent increased risk of death from any cause and about double the risk of death from a heart attack. Higher sodium consumption was also correlated with increased total mortality.

POTASSIUM-RICH DIET PERKS

Potassium-rich diets have been shown to have perks. Studies suggest they:

- **Boost your mood.** Balancing potassium and sodium intake may have mood-boosting benefits, according to a 2008 study published in the *British Journal of Nutrition*. Researchers randomly assigned middle-aged men and women to a low-sodium, high-potassium diet or to a moderate-sodium, high-calcium diet for four weeks after a two-week control diet. Those who followed the high-potassium, low-sodium diet showed greater improvement in depression, tension, vigor and overall mood compared to those who followed the moderate-sodium, high-calcium diet.

- **Benefit your bones.** In a study published in *Osteoporosis International* in 2009, researchers found that among 266 postmenopausal elderly women, those with the highest potassium levels had significantly higher bone mineral density measures at one and/or five years later, compared with those who had the lowest potassium levels. The researchers suggested that increasing the consumption of potassium-rich foods may play a role in preventing osteoporosis. A review that appeared in the *Journal of Nutrition* in 2008 also suggested that a potassium-rich, bicarbonate-rich diet (one rich in fruits and vegetables) can benefit bone health.

- **Maintain muscle mass.** In a review article published in *Proceedings of the Nutrition Society* in 2012, the authors posited that fruits and vegetables may protect against muscle loss because of their potassium content.

Because your kidneys usually excrete excess potassium, including too much potassium in your diet is seldom a problem. But extremely high intakes can lead to cardiac arrest and even death. Those who have kidney problems or who take potassium supplements are especially vulnerable to the damaging effects of too much potassium, so be sure to consult with a health-care provider before taking a potassium supplement or any other supplement. (See Appendix C for daily recommended intakes and upper limits for potassium.)

Potassium-Rich Foods

Here you'll find food sources that provide at least 10 percent of the Daily Value* (3,500 milligrams) of potassium.

Food	Portion	Potassium (mg)	Daily Value (%)**
Potatoes, baked	1 potato	1081	31
Spinach, fresh, cooked	1 cup	839	24
Prunes	1 cup	796	23
Prune juice, canned	1 cup	707	20
Sweet potatoes, baked	1 potato	694	20
Halibut, Atlantic or Pacific, cooked	4 ounces	599	17
Tuna, yellowfin, cooked	4 ounces	597	17
Yogurt, plain, nonfat	1 cup	579	17
Spinach, frozen, cooked	1 cup	574	16
Mushrooms, white, cooked	1 cup	555	16
Tomato puree, canned, without salt added	1/2 cup	549	16
Yogurt, plain, low-fat	1 cup	531	15
Beets, cooked	1 cup	519	15
Potatoes, boiled	1 cup	515	15
Rainbow trout, farmed, cooked	4 ounces	511	15
Pumpkin, canned, without salt	1 cup	505	14
Brussels sprouts, cooked	1 cup	495	14
Squash, winter, all varieties, cooked	1 cup	494	14
Soybeans, green and mature	1/2 cup	485	14
Artichokes, globe or French, cooked	1 cup	480	14
Lima beans, mature seeds, cooked	1/2 cup	478	14
Salmon, sockeye, cooked	4 ounces	463	13
Broccoli, fresh or frozen, cooked	1 cup	457	13

continued on page 104

Food	Portion	Potassium (mg)	Daily Value (%)**
Orange juice, chilled (includes from concentrate)	1 cup	443	13
Cucumber, with peel, raw	1 large cucumber	442	13
Cantaloupe	1 cup	427	12
Collards, frozen, cooked	1 cup	427	12
Tomatoes, red, raw	1 cup	427	12
Chocolate milk, low-fat	1 cup	425	12
Bananas	1 banana	422	12
Kale, frozen, cooked	1 cup	417	12
Grapefruit juice, white or pink	1 cup	400	11
Haddock, cooked	4 ounces	397	11
Honeydew melon	1 cup	388	11
Peas, edible pods, boiled	1 cup	384	11
Milk, nonfat	1 cup	382	11
Pinto beans, mature seeds, cooked	½ cup	373	11
Carrots, raw or cooked	1 cup	367	10
Turnip greens, frozen, cooked	1 cup	367	10
Lentils, mature seeds, cooked	½ cup	366	10
Red kidney beans, mature seeds, cooked	½ cup	357	10
Split peas, mature seeds, cooked	½ cup	355	10
Navy beans, mature seeds, cooked	½ cup	354	10

*Foods that provide 10 to 19 percent of the Daily Value of a nutrient are good sources. Foods that provide at least 20 percent of the Daily Value of a nutrient are excellent sources.

**Daily Value percentages are rounded to the nearest whole number.

Source: U.S. Department of Agriculture, Agricultural Research Service. 2012. USDA National Nutrient Database for Standard Reference, Release 25. Nutrient Data Laboratory Home Page, www.ars.usda.gov/nutrientdata.

MAGNESIUM

Magnesium has many important roles in the body. In addition to playing a vital role in bone formation (along with calcium and phosphorus), magnesium:

- Supports metabolism as a player in countless metabolic reactions, works with hundreds of enzymes and travels with adenosine triphosphate (ATP)—the key energy source for cells—to help it perform its crucial functions.

- Maintains nerve and muscle function, including that of the heart muscle.

- Helps turn carbohydrates and fat into fuel and facilitates the production of important proteins and genetic material, including DNA.

- Helps regulate levels of other minerals, including potassium, sodium and calcium, to support important body functions and maintain a fluid balance in the blood and cells.

There's also evidence that magnesium can help maintain healthy blood sugar and blood pressure levels, and support a healthy immune system.

HOW LOW CAN YOU GO?

Although a magnesium deficiency is rare, having low levels of magnesium in your diet and in your body can leave you feeling tired, weak, irritable or anxious, and can cause muscle cramps and even loss of sleep. A magnesium deficiency also can contribute to low blood levels of potassium. Low intakes and levels of magnesium can move you farther away from the 7 Pillars of Vitality. Here's why.

THEY ADD HUFF TO YOUR PUFF

There's evidence that too little magnesium can make your workouts that much harder. In a study published in the *Journal of Nutrition* in 2002, researchers set out to determine how a low magnesium intake affected exercise performance. They gave ten postmeno-pausal women a diet with adequate magnesium for five weeks. Then they gave the women a diet with only half the magnesium for ninety-three days. Finally, the women followed an adequate magnesium diet for another forty-nine days. At the end of each dietary phase, the subjects used an exercise bicycle that was measured and monitored.

The researchers found that the women had lower magnesium levels, lower red blood cell counts (which means they used more oxygen during their physical activity) and higher heart rates after having followed the low-magnesium diet. In a 2008 article in *Magnesium Research*, the authors suggested that eating too little dietary magnesium, coupled with strenuous or prolonged exercise, not only diminishes performance but also can lower immunity and increase the risk of infections, such as the common cold, perhaps by boosting inflammation.

THEY PUT YOU AT RISK FOR DEPRESSION

A few studies have linked low magnesium levels with a greater risk of depression. A 2012 study published in *Nutrition Journal* found an association between a low dietary intake of magnesium and depression, and a study that appeared in *Archives of Medical Research* in 2007 showed an association between low serum levels of magnesium and depression. But the news isn't all grim. Some studies suggest that getting enough magnesium helps beat the blues. In a study published in *Biological Trace Element Research* in 2012, researchers found an inverse relationship between magnesium intake and depressive symptoms in 402 men and women in their thirties. And in a review in *Nutritional Neuroscience* in 2012, researchers determined that higher dietary intakes of magnesium were linked with reduced depression symptoms. Researchers concluded that magnesium seems to be an effective treatment for depression.

Magnesium-Rich Foods

Here you'll find food sources that provide at least 10 percent of the Daily Value* (400 milligrams) of magnesium. (Any mention of brand-name items should not be construed as an implied endorsement.)

Food	Portion	Magnesium (mg)	Daily Value (%)**
Spinach, fresh or frozen, cooked	1 cup	157	39
Brazil nuts	1 ounce	107	27
Kellogg's Raisin Bran	1 cup	77	19
Almonds	1 ounce	76	19

Food	Portion	Magnesium (mg)	Daily Value (%)**
Cashews, dry-roasted	1 ounce	74	19
Okra, frozen, cooked	1 cup	74	19
Soybeans, mature, cooked	1/2 cup	74	19
Crab, Alaskan king, cooked	4 ounces	72	18
Artichokes, globe or French, cooked	1 cup	71	18
Pine nuts, dried	1 ounce	71	18
Mixed nuts, dry-roasted	1 ounce	64	16
Oats, regular and quick or instant, cooked with water	1 packet/ 1 cup	63	16
Shredded wheat cereal	2 biscuits	61	15
Black beans, mature seeds, cooked	1/2 cup	60	15
Bulgur, cooked	1 cup	58	15
Okra, fresh, cooked	1 cup	58	15
Potatoes, baked	1 potato	57	14
Pumpkin, canned	1 cup	56	14
Sweet potatoes, canned	1 cup	56	14
Kellogg's All-Bran Complete Wheat Flakes	3/4 cup	55	14
Collards, frozen, cooked	1 cup	51	13
Peanuts, dry-roasted	1 ounce	50	13
Espresso	2 fluid ounces	48	12
Navy beans, mature seeds, cooked	1/2 cup	48	12
Kellogg's Frosted Mini-Wheats	1 cup	47	12
Hazelnuts (filberts)	1 ounce	46	12
Great Northern beans, mature seeds, cooked	1/2 cup	45	11
Parsnips	1 cup	45	11

continued on page 108

Food	Portion	Magnesium (mg)	Daily Value (%)**
Walnuts, English	1 ounce	45	11
Cheerios	1 cup	43	11
Cowpeas (black-eyed peas), mature seeds, cooked	½ cup	43	11
Pinto beans, mature seeds, cooked	½ cup	43	11
Squash, summer, all varieties, cooked	1 cup	43	11
Yogurt, plain, nonfat	1 cup	43	11
Turnip greens, frozen, cooked	1 cup	43	11
Brown rice, long-grain, cooked	½ cup	42	10
Crab, blue, canned	4 ounces	42	10
Peas, edible pods, boiled	1 cup	42	10
Spaghetti, whole-wheat, cooked	1 cup	42	10
Lima beans, mature seeds, cooked	½ cup	41	10
Salmon, sockeye, cooked	4 ounces	41	10
Red kidney beans, mature seeds, cooked	½ cup	40	10

*Foods that provide 10 to 19 percent of the Daily Value of a nutrient are good sources. Foods that provide at least 20 percent of the Daily Value of a nutrient are excellent sources.

**Daily Value percentages are rounded to the nearest whole number.

Source: U.S. Department of Agriculture, Agricultural Research Service. 2012. USDA National Nutrient Database for Standard Reference, Release 25. Nutrient Data Laboratory Home Page, www.ars.usda.gov/nutrientdata.

CALCIUM

More abundant than any other mineral, calcium plays significant roles in your body. Alongside vitamin D and phosphorus, it helps form and maintain strong bones and teeth, which is especially critical for women, who are at risk for low bone mass and osteoporosis. Calcium also helps muscles contract and blood vessels relax and constrict.

And it transmits nerve impulses and helps enzymes and hormones function properly. Several studies have found that higher calcium intakes are associated with lower body weight (and lower body fat), improved blood lipids, a lower risk of type 2 diabetes and hypertension, and better metabolic health.

Like potassium, calcium is a "nutrient of concern" because many of us fail to meet recommended intake levels (see Appendix C for recommended calcium intake). You may be at risk for too little calcium if you avoid dairy products and don't get enough calcium from nondairy sources. Skimping on calcium takes its toll on your vitality in so many ways. There's evidence that it can:

- **Harm your bones.** In a study published in the *Journal of Bone and Mineral Research* in 2012, researchers looked at more than 4,662 Korean adults aged fifty and older who had low dietary calcium intakes, and found that calcium intake was a significant determinant of bone mineral density at both higher and lower vitamin D levels.

- **Hurt your muscles.** A study that appeared in the *Endocrine Journal* in 2009 found a strong inverse association between daily dietary calcium intake and muscle loss in non-obese older Korean adults. The association was particularly strong in adults with the highest calcium intakes versus those with the lowest intakes.

- **Lead to depression.** In a study published in *Nutrition in Research and Practice* in 2012, researchers analyzed three-day dietary records in 105 women aged forty-one to fifty-seven years and found that low daily intakes (less than five hundred milligrams) of dietary calcium (and calcium specifically from animal foods) was associated with more depression.

- **Cause disease.** A review article published in *Nutrients* in 2013 found that a low habitual calcium intake contributes to the risk of several chronic diseases, including osteoporosis, colorectal and breast cancer, and hypertension.

Calcium May Give PMS the Boot

On the plus side, there's some evidence that a high intake of calcium and vitamin D may help prevent the *real* PMS, premenstrual syndrome. In a study published in the *Archives of Internal Medicine* in 2005, researchers examined data for more than three thousand women aged twenty-seven to forty-four over ten years and determined that those with the highest daily intake of calcium from food had a 30 percent *lower* risk of developing PMS than those with the lowest intake. For vitamin D intake from foods, women with the highest intake had a 31 percent lower risk of PMS than women with the lowest intake.

Calcium-Rich Foods

Here you'll find food sources that provide at least 10 percent of the Daily Value* (1,000 milligrams) of calcium. (Any mention of brand-name items should not be construed as an implied endorsement.)

Food	Portion	Calcium (mg)	Daily Value (%)**
Raisin bran cereal	1 cup	1038	104
General Mills Total Whole Grain	1 cup	1000	100
Yogurt, plain, nonfat	1 cup	452	45
Sardines, Atlantic, canned in oil, drained, with bones	4 ounces	433	43
Yogurt, plain, low-fat	1 cup	415	42
Collards, fresh or frozen, cooked	1 cup	357	36
Rhubarb, frozen, cooked	1 cup	348	35
Ricotta cheese, part-skim	½ cup	335	34
Milk, low-fat	1 cup	305	31
Milk, nonfat	1 cup	299	30
Spinach, frozen, cooked	1 cup	291	29
Chocolate milk, low-fat	1 cup	290	29
Buttermilk, low-fat	1 cup	284	28
Salmon, pink, canned	4 ounces	244	24

Food	Portion	Calcium (mg)	Daily Value (%)**
Swiss cheese	1 ounce	224	22
Provolone cheese	1 ounce	214	21
Cowpeas (black-eyed peas), immature seeds, cooked	1/2 cup	211	21
Mozzarella cheese, part skim	1 ounce	207	21
Cheddar cheese	1 ounce	204	20
Muenster cheese	1 ounce	203	20
Turnip greens, cooked	1 cup	197	20
Kale, frozen, cooked	1 cup	179	18
Shrimp, canned	4 ounces	164	16
Tofu, firm, prepared with calcium, sulfate and magnesium chloride (nigari)	1/4 block (about 3 ounces)	163	16
Cabbage, Chinese (bok choy), cooked	1 cup	158	16
Blue cheese	1 ounce	150	15
Camembert cheese	1 ounce	147	15
Mozzarella cheese, whole milk	1 ounce	143	14
Oats, instant, fortified, plain, prepared with water	1 packet	142	14
Feta cheese	1 ounce	140	14
Okra, frozen or fresh, cooked	1 cup	136	14
Soybeans, green, cooked	1/2 cup	131	13
Cheerios	1 cup	122	12
Cheddar or Colby cheese, low-fat	1 ounce	118	12
Kellogg's All-Bran cereal	1/2 cup	117	12
Crab, blue, canned	4 ounces	105	10
Mustard greens, cooked	1 cup	104	10
White beans, mature seeds, canned	1/2 cup	96	10

continued on page 112

Calcium, Potassium and Magnesium, Oh My!

When you're super busy, it's hard to think of how you're possibly going to get potassium, magnesium, calcium and other vital minerals into your diet. Fortunately, you can get all these Vital Nutrients (and then some) in no time by whipping up some simple smoothies created by registered dietitian and chef Michelle Dudash, author of *Clean Eating for Busy Families*.

Basic ingredients: $1/2$ cup liquid (such as milk or orange juice) + $1/4$ to $1/2$ cup creamy ingredient (such as yogurt, banana, beans or nut butter) + 1 cup chopped fruit + 4 ice cubes + $1/8$ teaspoon flavoring (such as vanilla extract or cinnamon) or more to taste + 1 teaspoon honey or agave nectar, only if needed for taste.

Directions: Pour liquids and creamy ingredients into the blender, followed by the solid ingredients. Cover and puree on low, working up to high speed, until smooth, about 30 to 60 seconds. Enjoy immediately.

Try one of these combos:

Go Berry with Banana: $1/2$ cup low-fat milk, $1/4$ cup vanilla yogurt, $1/2$ cup strawberries (halved), 1 small banana (quartered), $1/8$ teaspoon vanilla extract and 1 teaspoon honey.

Get a Zing from Sneaky Greens: $1/2$ cup orange juice, $1/2$ cup low-fat Greek vanilla yogurt, 1 cup blueberries, $1/2$ cup baby spinach and 1 teaspoon sliced fresh ginger.

Get Your Zen On: $1/2$ cup cold unsweetened green tea, $1/2$ cup vanilla yogurt + 1 tablespoon almond butter, 1 cup chopped mango, 2 teaspoons lemon juice and 1 teaspoon honey.

Like a Pina Colada: $1/2$ cup coconut milk, $1/4$ cup low-fat cottage cheese, $3/4$ cup frozen pineapple chunks, 1 banana (quartered) and $1/8$ teaspoon cinnamon.

Dream in Creamy Orange: $1/2$ cup almond milk, $1/2$ banana (quartered), 1 orange (chopped), 1 tablespoon almond butter and $1/8$ teaspoon cinnamon.

Do I Need to Eat Dairy Foods?

Dairy foods—especially low-fat and nonfat milk and yogurt—provide lots of highly absorbable calcium and other key nutrients, including protein, vitamin D, potassium, phosphorus, magnesium, vitamins A and D, vitamin B$_{12}$ and riboflavin (see Glossary to learn more about these Vital Nutrients). Eating dairy foods is linked with improved bone health (and reduced osteoporosis risk), as well as lower blood pressure and a reduced risk of cardiovascular disease and type 2 diabetes. Current Dietary Guidelines for Americans recommend three daily dairy servings. But if you don't like the taste of dairy or avoid it because of lactose intolerance or for other reasons, you can get calcium from fortified soy beverages and foods that are naturally calcium rich, such as beans, leafy greens and fish (see Calcium-Rich Foods on page 110). Calcium-fortified orange juice and other fortified foods also provide calcium, though it's usually not as readily absorbed as that in dairy foods. Avoiding dairy altogether can also leave you short of vitamin D and other valuable nutrients. Be sure to eat sardines with the bones, tuna, eggs and fortified cereals to ensure you're getting enough calcium. And if you know you won't eat any or enough dairy or other calcium-rich foods to meet your needs, discuss supplementation with your doctor or registered dietitian so you don't fall short on this Vital Nutrient.

SODIUM

We all need a relatively small amount of sodium in our daily diet. It's an essential mineral that works with other minerals, primarily potassium and chloride, to maintain fluid balance in the body. Sodium also plays a role in regulating blood pressure, helps muscles—including the heart—contract and relax, and transmits nerve impulses. But while consuming too little sodium or losing too much through exercise, for example, can put you at risk for low sodium levels, which can cause a headache, nausea, dizziness, fatigue, muscle cramps and even fainting, most of us consume far too much sodium. National survey data suggests that, on average, women consume about 3,000 milligrams of sodium daily—that's more than the 2,300 milligrams recommended daily and *twice* the 1,500 milligrams recommended for adults who are aged fifty-one or older, who are African American or who have hypertension, diabetes or chronic kidney disease. Even if we do not use our salt shakers, we may still be consuming too much sodium. Many of the packaged, processed foods we rely on daily are loaded with sodium. And a single restaurant entrée or a fast-food meal can easily supply an entire day's worth of sodium.

Consuming too much sodium can have a variety of vitality-busting effects. Besides making us feel bloated, too much sodium can:

- **Harm your heart.** A higher sodium intake usually contributes to higher blood pressure levels and in some people can lead to hypertension—a risk factor for heart attack and stroke. In a study published in *CNS Neuroscience and Therapeutics* in 2012, researchers reviewed twelve studies with almost 226,000 participants, who were followed for three to nineteen years, and found that a high salt intake was associated with stroke risk.

- **Compromise calcium.** Several studies suggest that a higher sodium intake may lead to increased excretion of calcium and lower bone mineral density. For example, a study that appeared in *Nutrients* in 2011 found that a higher dietary sodium intake was associated with greater calcium excretion and lower hip bone density in young women with a low calcium intake. In his review article about dietary sodium and osteoporosis published in the *Journal of the American College of Nutrition* in 2006, Robert P. Heaney, MD, suggested that sodium elevates urinary calcium excretion, and that when calcium intake is less than adequate, bone loss can occur.

Too much sodium can also lead to dehydration if you don't drink enough water; this can be a problem, particularly if you work out hard. Although excess sodium usually can be excreted by healthy kidneys, people with impaired kidney function or those who overdo it on calcium may not be able to excrete the excess sodium. This can contribute to facial swelling or swelling in the extremities.

What's the Difference between Salt and Sodium?

Table salt is made of sodium and another mineral, chloride. Chloride, a key part of hydrochloric acid (gastric juice, which helps you digest and absorb nutrients), works with sodium and potassium to regulate water balance. It also supports nerve and immune function. Forty percent of salt is sodium and the other 60 percent is chloride. If you want to know how many milligrams of salt a packaged food contains, multiply the milligrams of sodium per serving listed on the Nutrition Facts panel by 2.5. For example, if a condiment has 300 milligrams of sodium per serving, then it has 750 milligrams of salt (300 x 2.5 = 750 milligrams of salt).

SEVEN TIPS TO SLASH SODIUM

With sodium so abundant in our food supply, we need to make a real effort to cut back. While restaurants and food manufacturers are stepping up to the plate to help us reduce our sodium intake with improved disclosure on menu boards and "reduced-sodium" and "low-sodium" items, it's really up to us to lower our sodium intake. Here are seven simple ways to painlessly slash sodium without sacrificing taste:

1. **See where sodium lurks.** If you eat packaged foods, read the labels to see which items have the most sodium. For example, most ready-to-eat breakfast cereals have a few hundred milligrams of sodium. Reduce sodium here by swapping your favorite cereal for virtually sodium-free shredded wheat. You can also replace half your usual portion of cereal with shredded wheat to cut your sodium intake from cereal in half.

2. **Can up.** Be mindful of the sodium that lurks in canned vegetables, canned legumes (beans and peas) and canned soups, including tomato soup. When possible, choose canned foods that are labeled "sodium-free" or have "no sodium" (less than 5 milligrams of sodium and contain no sodium chloride ingredients), "very low sodium" (35 milligrams of sodium or less), "low sodium" (140 milligrams of sodium or less) or "reduced or less sodium" (at least 25 percent less sodium than the regular product). Rinsing canned vegetables, including beans, can also help you significantly slash sodium (by as much as 40 percent, according to one study).

3. **Swap your salad dressing.** Creamy Italian, Caesar and other types of bottled dressings are notorious for their high-sodium content. Many, especially low-fat and nonfat options, also have added sugar to boost flavor. Opt instead for homemade vinaigrette, made with olive oil and balsamic vinegar, which together provide heart-healthy fats and phytochemicals. If you do use salty salad dressing, stick to two tablespoons or less, and dip your fork into it "on the side" instead of pouring it over your salad greens.

4. **Cap your add-ons and condiments**. Even seemingly healthful dietary additions, such as olives, pickles, store-bought guacamole or hummus, salsa, ketchup, mustard and tomato sauce, are packed with sodium—even in relatively small portions. Follow the one-to-two tablespoon rule (or have just a few pickle slices or olives) for such add-ons.

5. **Use (or choose) better prep methods**. When cooking at home, add no-salt seasonings (like herbs and spices) in place of salt. And when you do use salt, add it in tiny amounts after the meal is cooked (rather than during cooking, when the taste gets diluted). When ordering at a restaurant, choose foods that are grilled, baked or lightly sautéed, rather than breaded or fried. You can also ask that your food be prepared without added salt.

6. **Snack smarter**. Did you know that ounce for ounce, pretzels have more than twice the sodium as potato chips (359 vs. 136 milligrams, respectively)? Salted mixed nuts have even less (about 98 milligrams per ounce). Choose nuts and other "reduced" or "low-sodium" bagged and boxed snack options over high-sodium ones more often. You can also make your own popcorn with a little oil and low- or no-sodium toppings (see Chapter 3 and Chapter 14 for more ideas).

7. **Go for produce.** Fill up on fresh fruits and vegetables, which are naturally low in sodium and rich in potassium. Including produce in every meal and snack can also fill you up, which can indirectly help you reduce your intake of salty, fatty or sugary fare.

Get in Tune with Your PMS-C

- Load up on potassium-rich foods, including produce, often. Excellent sources include baked potatoes, cooked spinach, prunes and prune juice, and sweet potatoes.

- Vary your diet to get a magnesium boost. Foods such as ready-to-eat whole-grain cereals, oats, nuts and beans are good to excellent sources of this Vital Nutrient.

- Consume calcium daily by choosing low-fat or nonfat yogurt, milk and cheese; fish with bones (such as sardines or salmon); beans; and soybeans and soy foods (such as tofu).

- Slash your sodium intake by eating more fresh foods and fewer processed and packaged foods; using herbs and spices (see Chapter 8) when preparing, cooking or eating food; and reading labels when food shopping to see where sodium lurks.

PROTEST THE RADICALS WITH ANTIOXIDANTS

Here's an easy fix. Adding fruits and vegetables to your meals, sprinkling foods with herbs and spices, and yes, even enjoying some chocolate and sipping tea will provide your body with nutrients and plant chemicals—many of which act as antioxidants. These nutrients and antioxidants protect your skin, your organs and your entire body from the ravages caused by a buildup of free radicals and other harmful chemicals that you're exposed to on a daily basis.

Oxygen is a true "frenemy." You need it to live, when you breathe, exercise or eat. But when your body breaks it down for immediate energy (or stores it for later use), it generates highly reactive, unstable molecules called free radicals. Free radicals also are created when you're exposed to environmental elements, such as radiation and ultraviolet light from the sun, and to contaminants, such as cigarette smoke, pesticides and other toxins found in food and water, and even when you're stressed.

Having some of these free radicals present in your body is actually beneficial because they protect you from germs and infections that can lead to colds or diseases, and they help nerve cells in your brain communicate with one another. Normally, your body's antioxidant defense system protects against cell damage caused by free radicals. But chronic exposure to high levels of free radicals can overwhelm your body's natural defenses and contribute to a condition called oxidative stress—a state in which cells of the body, including carbohydrates, fats, proteins and even DNA, the body's basic genetic material, are vulnerable to injury. Researchers believe that oxidative stress ages us, resulting in wrinkles, saggy skin and psychological stress. Oxidative stress has also been linked with the onset and progression of heart disease, cancer and Alzheimer's disease; with inflammatory conditions, such as rheumatoid arthritis; and with depressed immunity, which makes us vulnerable to colds, the flu and infection. It's clear that oxidative stress can really put the squeeze on your vitality.

While the cells in your body naturally produce some antioxidants, the best way to more fully protect yourself against the ravages of free radicals and oxidative stress (a marker for aging) is by consuming a diet that's rich in essential antioxidant nutrients, such as vitamin C (see Gimme a C! on page 122), vitamin E and the mineral selenium. (See the Glossary for more on these Vital Nutrients.) The good news is that you can arm yourself with fruits, vegetables and other plant foods that provide these and other antioxidant compounds. Many of these compounds, called phytochemicals, protect us in several different ways. According to Jeffrey Blumberg, PhD, director of the Antioxidants Research Laboratory at the Jean Mayer USDA Human Nutrition Research Center on Aging, although many phytochemicals do not directly squash free radicals the way vitamin C, vitamin E and selenium do, they do enhance our defenses by stimulating our cells to synthesize enzymes that act as antioxidants and detoxifiers and inhibit signals that promote inflammation.

Antioxidants are found in a wide variety of foods, including whole grains (see Chapter 3), nuts (see Chapter 4), fruits, vegetables, herbs and spices, and even chocolate. Tea is another great source of antioxidants, and I go into more detail about that in Chapter 9.

FRUITS AND VEGETABLES

You've always heard how important it is to eat fruits and vegetables, and eating lots of produce is essential to looking and feeling your best. Besides being a key source of dietary fiber and potassium, which many of us don't get enough of on a daily basis, fruits and vegetables are packed with many other nutrients we need, including vitamin C, a key antioxidant nutrient (see Gimme a C! on page 122), folate, magnesium, vitamin A and vitamin K (see Vital Nutrients in Fruits below and Vital Nutrients in Vegetables on page 121, and refer to the Glossary to learn more about these Vital Nutrients).

Vital Nutrients in Fruits

Here are some of the fruits that are good (G) and excellent (E) sources of fiber and key vitamins and minerals.*

Fruit	Fiber	Vitamin A	Vitamin K	Vitamin C	Vitamin B$_6$	Folate	Potassium	Selenium	Copper	Mangnese
Apple (1 medium)	G			G						
Banana (1 medium)	G			G	E		G			G
Blackberries (1 cup)	E		E	E					G	E
Blueberries (1 cup)	G		E	E						E
Cantaloupe (1 cup)		E		E			G			
Grapefruit (1 medium)	G	E		E			G			
Grapes, red/green (32)			E							
Guava (1 cup diced)	E	E		E		E	G		G	G
Orange (1 large)	G			E		G				
Papaya (1 cup)	G	E		E		G				
Peach (1 large)	G	G		G						
Pineapple (1 cup chunks)				E						E
Raspberries (1 cup)	E		G	E				G		E
Strawberries (1 cup)	G			E						E

*Foods that provide 10 to 19 percent of the Daily Value of a nutrient are good sources. Foods that provide at least 20 percent of the Daily Value of a nutrient are excellent sources.

Source: U.S. Department of Agriculture, Agricultural Research Service. 2012. USDA National Nutrient Database for Standard Reference, Release 25. Nutrient Data Laboratory Home Page, www.ars.usda.gov/nutrientdata.

Vital Nutrients in Vegetables

Here are some of the vegetables that are good (G) and excellent (E) sources of fiber and key vitamins and minerals.*

Vegetable	Fiber	Vitamin A	Vitamin E	Vitamin K	Vitamin C	Thiamine	Riboflavin	Niacin	Pantothenic Acid	Vitamin B$_6$	Folate	Potassium	Calcium	Phosphorus	Magnesium	Manganese	Iron	Selenium	Copper
Artichoke (1/2 cup cooked)	E			E	E						E	G		G	G				G
Asparagus (1 cup cooked)	G	E		E	E	G	G				E	G						G	G
Broccoli (1 cup cooked)	E	E		E	E		G			G	E	G	G	G					
Brussels sprouts (1 cup cooked)	G	E		E	E	G				G	E	G					G		
Butternut squash (1/2 cup cooked)	E	E			E					G		G			G				
Carrots (1 cup sliced)	G	E		E	G							G							
Chard (1 cup cooked)	G	E		E	E							E	G		E		E		G
Kale (1 cup cooked)	G	E		E	E										E				G
Mushrooms, white (1 cup cooked)	G				G		E	E	E	G				G			G	E	E
Onion (1/2 cup cooked)	G				G					G									

continued on page 122

Vegetable	Fiber	Vitamin A	Vitamin E	Vitamin K	Vitamin C	Thiamine	Riboflavin	Niacin	Pantothenic Acid	Vitamin B6	Folate	Potassium	Calcium	Phosphorus	Magnesium	Manganese	Iron	Selenium	Copper
Spinach (1 cup cooked)	G	E	G	E	E	G	E			E	E	E	E	G	E		E	G	G
Tomato (1 cup chopped, raw)		E		G	E							G							

*Foods that provide 10 to 19 percent of the Daily Value of a nutrient are good sources. Foods that provide at least 20 percent of the Daily Value of a nutrient are excellent sources.

Source: U.S. Department of Agriculture, Agricultural Research Service. 2012. USDA National Nutrient Database for Standard Reference, Release 25. Nutrient Data Laboratory Home Page, www.ars.usda.gov/nutrientdata.

Gimme a C!

Vitamin C, a water-soluble vitamin, is an antioxidant nutrient that helps protect skin and body cells from free-radical damage. It facilitates the production of collagen, the body's main structural protein, which holds the skin, the bones and other tissues together, supports healthy gums and plays a key role in wound healing. A study published in 2007 in the *American Journal of Clinical Nutrition* found evidence that consuming more vitamin C–rich foods can contribute to fewer wrinkles and less dry skin in middle-aged women. Vitamin C also supports a healthy immune system and helps your body absorb iron from food. It's also involved in the creation of norepinephrine, a chemical in the brain that affects mood. To enjoy the benefits of vitamin C–and other potent nutrients and plant chemi-cals–choose several of these vitamin C-rich fruits and vegetables weekly: broccoli, Brussels sprouts, cauliflower, green peppers, guava, kale, kohlrabi, orange juice, oranges, papaya, potatoes, sweet red peppers, sweet potatoes and low-sodium tomato juice.

Fruits and vegetables also boast a wide variety of phytochemicals, many of which act as antioxidants. These include carotenoids (beta-carotene, lycopene, lutein and zeaxanthan), flavonoids (anthocyanadins, flavanols, flavonones, proanthocyanidins and quercetin) and phenols (caffeic acid, ferulic acid and resveratrol). To reap all the benefits provided by fruits and vegetables, it's essential to eat a wide variety of colorful options.

VITAL BENEFITS OF FRUITS AND VEGETABLES

Eating fruits and vegetables has many perks. Here are just some of the recent findings that will leave you saying, "Please pass the produce."

THEY IMPROVE APPEARANCE

There's proof that eating your fruits and vegetables makes you not only feel better but look pretty too. In a study published in *PloS One* in 2012, researchers investigated the effects of fruit and vegetable intake on skin color. Dietary intake and skin color were recorded at the start of the study and three and six weeks after for thirty-five white male and female college students. Increased fruit and vegetable consumption over six weeks improved the color and appearance of skin by increasing its yellowness and redness, likely because of the carotenoids that fruits and vegetables contain. Researchers also asked twenty-four undergraduates to rate computer-generated images of people who ate different amounts of fruits and vegetables by how healthy or attractive they looked. Based on the findings, the researchers concluded that having about 2¼ to 2½ cups of produce daily may contribute to the healthier appearance of skin or enhance attractiveness.

THEY PROMOTE SKIN HEALTH

A review published in *Nutrients* in 2010 provides evidence that besides making your skin look more radiant, consuming a diet rich in phytonutrients—many of which act as antioxidants, such as alpha-tocopherol (a form of vitamin E), flavonoids, beta-carotene, lycopene and lutein—protects the skin and the entire body from UV damage, which contributes to oxidative stress, inflammation, wrinkling and skin cancer.

THEY PROTECT YOUR WAISTLINE

Fruits and vegetables are loaded with water to keep you hydrated. Studies also suggest that consuming water from foods like fruits, vegetables and cooked grains is far more effective at filling you up than drinking water. Studies by Barbara Rolls, PhD, and her colleagues at the Pennsylvania State University suggest that incorporating fruits and vegetables into your diet—especially in place of more high-calorie foods—can help you achieve and maintain a healthier body weight (and possibly lose weight) by reducing the energy density of your diet, filling you up and helping you feel more satisfied, and decreasing your overall calorie intake.

THEY PROTECT AGAINST CHRONIC DISEASE

In a review that appeared in the *European Journal of Nutrition* in 2012, researchers found convincing evidence that increasing fruit and vegetable intake reduces the risk of hypertension, CHD and stroke. They also found evidence that consuming fruits and vegetables may lower cancer risk and that the intake of those foods is inversely related to cancer risk. In addition, the researchers suggested that eating more produce may prevent weight gain and indirectly reduce type 2 diabetes risk. They also concluded that eating fruits and vegetables may lower the risk of some eye diseases, dementia and osteoporosis.

THEY PROTECT YOUR BRAIN

In a study published in the *Journal of Nutrition, Health and Aging* in 2012, German researchers reviewed nine studies that included more than forty-four thousand participants to determine the link between fruit and vegetable intake and the risk of cognitive decline or dementia. Five out of six studies concluded that a higher intake of vegetables, but not fruit, was associated with a lower risk of dementia and slower rates of cognitive decline. Three other studies found similar results for combined fruit and vegetable intake. Another study, this one published in the *Journal of Alzheimer's Disease* in 2009, found that healthy adults between the ages of forty-five and 102 who had a high daily intake of fruits and vegetables had higher antioxidant levels, better cognitive performance and less oxidative stress than healthy adults who had a low intake. In a study that appeared in *Neurology* in 2005, Harvard researchers prospectively examined fruit and vegetable intake in relation to cognitive function and decline in more than thirteen thousand aging women. Those who consumed the most cruciferous vegetables (such as broccoli, kale and Brussels sprouts) showed slower cognitive decline compared with those who consumed the least. Those who consumed the most leafy green vegetables also experienced slower cognitive decline than those who consumed the least.

THEY HELP YOU AGE BETTER

Eating fruits and vegetables may be linked with healthy aging. A study published in the *Canadian Medical Association Journal* in 2012, which included 5,100 men and women aged forty-two to sixty-three, evaluated subjects' healthy behaviors, such as never smoking, moderate alcohol consumption, moderate physical activity at least 2½ hours a week or at least 1 hour per week of vigorous physical activity, and eating fruits and vegetables daily. "Successful aging" over a follow-up of more than sixteen years was defined as good cognitive, physical, respiratory and cardiovascular functioning and the absence of disability, mental health problems and chronic disease. Compared with subjects who engaged in no healthy behaviors, participants who engaged in all four healthy behaviors were 3.3 times more likely to age successfully, meaning that the more healthy behaviors you adopt, the better your chance of aging "successfully."

Vital Antioxidants: Flavonoids

According to a review published in the *Journal of Nutrition in Gerontology and Geriatrics* in 2012, flavonoids–phenolic antioxidants found in fruits and vegetables, herbs and spices, chocolate, essential oils, and beverages–have the most potential to promote bone health, besides calcium and vitamin D. The researchers cite epidemiological studies that suggest flavonoid consumption has a more positive impact on bone health than general fruit and vegetable consumption. The researchers speculate that the effects of flavonoids are due to their antioxidant capacity and possibly their anti-inflammatory properties, as well.

Do 'Em or Ditch 'Em?

Fruit and Vegetable Juices

I am a strong believer in "Food first, then juice." That's because, compared with juice, whole fruits and vegetables are packed with more fiber and Vital Nutrients and take longer to eat, so they make you feel full–two qualities that can make them a win-win health- and weight-wise. But small amounts of 100 percent fruit juices, such as orange, cranberry or grapefruit juice,* low- or no-sodium vegetable juices, and juices made at home using a combination of fruits, vegetables and no-sugar ingredients can be a great source

continued on page 126

of antioxidants, vitamins and minerals to help you meet your daily quota. For example, registered dietitian Lauren Slayton recommends a basic green juice made with four cups of kale, one cucumber, four celery stalks, one pear and a piece of peeled fresh ginger (the size of a quarter). Bottom line? Do 'em, but don't overdo 'em, and make sure to consume plenty of whole fruits and vegetables, too.

*Grapefruit juice should not be taken with certain blood pressure-lowering medications and some anti-anxiety or insomnia medications, so if you take any of these, be sure to consult with a doctor before you drink this juice.

Vital Veggies

Although all vegetables provide nutrients and other beneficial substances, cruciferous vegetables, including kale, collard greens, cabbage, Brussels sprouts, kohlrabi, broccoli, cauliflower and Chinese cabbage, are standouts for their antioxidant and anti-inflammatory benefits. Some studies suggest that these members of the Brassicaceae family (including Brussels sprouts, my favorite) may protect the heart and have anti-cancer properties. Choose several of these vital veggies each week to maximize their many antioxidant and other benefits.

TIPS TO FIT IN FRUITS AND VEGETABLES

Despite the perks of produce, many Americans fail to meet recommended intakes. Although current Dietary Guidelines for Americans recommend one and a half cups of fruit and two to two and a half cups of vegetables daily for most women, national survey data shows that most women eat less than one cup of fruit and one and a half cups of vegetables daily.

Fitting more fruits and vegetables into your diet does not have to feel like a chore. To start, set yourself up for success by keeping small amounts of fresh produce, canned and frozen vegetables (preferably those with no salt added), and unsweetened dried and canned fruit on hand. Keeping whole fresh fruit in a bowl on your kitchen counter or sliced fruit or berries in a glass or translucent bowl in your refrigerator will also remind you (and your spouse, partner and/or kids) to "help yourself." Pairing dried fruit with other antioxidant-rich foods, such as nuts and seeds and whole-grain cereal, provides an even healthier boost. Choosing one fruit or vegetable at every (or nearly every) meal or snacktime. Eating it first can help fill you up and leave less room for high-calorie, less nutritious food. Juice, either fruit or vegetable, can also be an option (see Do 'Em or Ditch 'Em: Fruit and Vegetable Juices on page 125) as long as you limit portions and eat plenty of whole fruits and vegetables.

HERBS, SPICES AND EVERYTHING NICE

Herbs and spices are potent sources of antioxidants. In a study published in *Nutrition Journal* in 2010, researchers reviewed 3,100 foods for their antioxidant content. The following herbs and spices (dried and ground) emerged as antioxidant all-stars, based on one hundred grams: clove, peppermint, allspice, cinnamon, oregano, thyme, sage, rosemary, saffron and tarragon. And an analysis of 1,120 food samples published in the *American Journal of Clinical Nutrition* in 2006 showed that several herbs and spices reigned supreme in terms of their antioxidant content. In particular, ground cloves, dried oregano, ground ginger, ground cinnamon, turmeric powder, dried basil and ground yellow mustard seeds boasted particularly high amounts of antioxidants, based on one hundred grams. Ground cloves ranked tenth out of the 1,113 foods examined, based on typical serving sizes. In both studies, dried herbs and spices, perhaps surprisingly, contained significantly more antioxidants than their fresh counterparts.

When it comes to your vitality, studies suggest that herbs and spices can be key players. According to a review by researchers at the Agricultural Research Service (ARS) of the USDA in 2012, herbs and spices appear to possess antioxidant, anti-inflammatory, antihypertensive (blood pressure–lowering) qualities, along with other beneficial health effects. Researchers posited that the polyphenols (plant chemicals) found in herbs and spices may, among their other benefits, protect the brain and cognitive function. In another review, this one published in the *World Journal of Gastroenterology* in 2010, the authors pointed to several studies that suggest that herbs and spices protect against infection by conferring antibacterial, antimicrobial and antifungal benefits.

Although we need far more data to determine whether herbs and spices have age-defying benefits, and how much you would need to eat in order to see these benefits, it's smart to use them to spice up your meals and snacks (like popcorn). And while they add little weight to your plate, herbs and spices can contribute meaningful amounts of antioxidants to your diet, especially if you use them to replace some or all of the salt you use while cooking or eating. See Top Herbs and Spices for Health to learn more about herbs and spices and how to incorporate them into your meals.

Top Herbs and Spices for Health

Herb or Spice	Description	Culinary Tips
Allspice	This cured, unripe berry from a tropical evergreen tree releases sweet, nutty flavors and aromas in both whole and ground form.	Use to flavor breads, desserts, cereals and coffee; pairs well with savory dishes, such as soups, sauces, grains and vegetables.
Anise	Related to the parsley family, small, curved aniseeds are famous for their licorice scent and flavor.	Use to flavor breads, cakes, and cookies; include in Indian and Middle Eastern stews.
Basil	This bright green leafy plant has a fresh, sweet herbal taste and aroma.	Use in salads, appetizers and side dishes, or in pesto over pasta and in sandwiches.
Bay leaves*	Those large leaves from the laurel tree lend a sharp, bitter taste to dishes.	Adds flavor to soups, stews, bean dishes and grilled vegetables.
Caraway seed	These seeds from the parsley family have a tangy, sweet taste.	Traditionally used in rye breads and cakes, they also accent cabbage dishes and soups.
Cardamom	Ground from seeds in the ginger family, this spice has a sweet, pungent flavor and smell.	Popular in Scandinavian baked breads and desserts, it's also good in coffee and in Indian dishes.
Celery seed	These dried seeds, which have a warm, slightly bitter flavor, are the very same seeds that celery grows from.	Delicious in soups, potato dishes, salad dressings and vegetable dishes.
Chervil	A lacy-leafed plant in the parsley family, this green herb has an anise-parsley flavor.	Use to flavor potatoes, grain pilafs, vinaigrettes, sauces and sautéed vegetables.
Chives	These thin, hollow leaves from a plant in the onion family produce a garlic-onion bite.	Use to flavor baked potatoes, steamed whole grains, and salads, or serve as a colorful garnish.
Cilantro	A leaf of the young coriander plant, it adds a citrus-parsley flavor.	Use to flavor Southwestern, Thai, Indian and Mexican foods.
Cinnamon	This dried, curled tree bark has a sweet, woody flavor in both stick and ground forms.	Add to fruits, baked desserts and breads, as well as savory Middle Eastern dishes.

Herb or Spice	Description	Culinary Tips
Cloves	These nail-shaped dried buds have a strong, sweet aroma and flavor in both whole and ground forms.	Traditionally used in baked goods and breads and with fruits; also pairs well with vegetable and bean dishes.
Coriander	This seed from the cilantro plant has a mild, lemon-sage taste and aroma in ground or whole forms.	Use with fruits and in baked goods, breads, chutneys, and Mediterranean and Asian dishes.
Cumin	Ground or whole, these small seeds lend a characteristic bitter yet warm flavor.	Good in Mexican, Indian and Middle Eastern dishes, as well as with vegetables and in chili.
Dill weed	This grassy, feathery plant has a clean, pungent taste.	Traditionally served with Russian, German and Scandinavian foods, it also accents potato dishes, salads and dips.
Fennel seed	The grayish, oval seeds of the fennel plant have a sweet anise flavor and aroma.	Great in pasta, grain and vegetable dishes, as well as vinaigrettes.
Garlic	This bulb, available fresh, minced, or dried and granulated, provides a distinctive, earthy aroma and bite.	Used in South African, Indian, French, Italian and Greek cooking; add to soups, pastas, marinades, dressings, grains and vegetables.
Ginger	A root that is sold fresh, pickled, dried and crystallized, it has a sweet, warm flavor and smell.	Popular in Asian and Indian sauces, stews and stir-fries; also good in beverages and baked goods.
Marjoram	Ground or whole, this herb in the mint family has a delicate, sweet quality.	Try it in stews, soups, salads and sauces, and with potatoes, beans and grains.
Mint	This green herb has a tangy, cool scent and taste.	Excellent in jams, savory dishes, beverages, salads and marinades, and with fruits.
Mustard seed	Whether whole or ground, these seeds from the Brassicaceae family add a spicy kick.	Use to flavor sauces, vinaigrettes, potato salad, and soups; make mustard by grinding mustard seeds with a bit of vinegar and water.
Nutmeg	This ground spice lends a sweet, woodsy quality to dishes.	Traditionally used with fruits and in pies and other baked goods; also suitable for soups and vegetable dishes.
Oregano	Both whole and ground forms of this herb in the mint family supply a warm woodsy aroma and taste.	Delicious in Italian and Mediterranean dishes; pairs with salads and tomato, pasta and grain dishes.
Parsley	A natural breath freshener, parsley boasts a clean, fresh flavor.	Add to soups, pasta dishes, salads and sauces; popular as a garnish.

continued on page 130

Herb or Spice	Description	Culinary Tips
Pepper, black or white	Cracked, whole or ground black or white pepper provides a sharp, hot flavor.	Seasons soups, stews, vegetable dishes, grains, pastas, beans, sauces and salads.
Pepper, red	The catchall term for all hot red pepper spices, such as cayenne, red pepper flakes and paprika, which provide a strong, hot bite.	Adds flavor to dishes such as beans, chilies, curries, sauces and marinades; a key ingredient in Mexican, Thai, Indian and Creole cooking.
Poppy seed	These dark, tiny seeds of the opium plant have a nutty taste and smell.	Use to flavor breads, pancakes, muffins, cakes, cookies and salad dressings, as well as noodle and vegetable dishes.
Rosemary	The needles of this herb possess an aromatic, piney quality.	Try it in vegetables, salads, vinaigrettes and pasta dishes.
Saffron	These precious red spice threads impart a golden hue and an earthy flavor and aroma.	A small pinch flavors rice dishes, risotto, stews, sauces and breads.
Sage	These cottony leaves supply a warm, astringent flavor and aroma in both whole and ground forms.	Traditionally paired with savory meat dishes; also enhances grains, breads, dressings, soups and pastas.
Tarragon	This green herb lends a slightly bittersweet aroma and flavor to dishes.	Delicious in sauces and marinades, it also flavors salads and bean dishes.
Thyme	Used ground or whole, these tiny gray-green leaves have a slightly minty taste.	Excellent in soups, tomato dishes and salads, and with vegetables.
Turmeric	The ground root boasts a bright orange-gold shade and a bold citrus-ginger flavor.	Essential in curry powder, it's most popular in Indian cooking; adds flavor to soups, beans and vegetables.
Vanilla (pure)	Derived from the long green pods of a tropical orchid, which are cured and steeped in alcohol, it has a sweet, perfumed taste.	Use in flavored beverages, plant-based dairy alternatives, sauces, fruits, breads and desserts.

*Discard the bay leaves, which have sharp edges and an unpleasant texture and pose a choking hazard, before you serve the dish.

Source: Adapted with permission from *The Plant-Powered Diet* (The Experiment, 2012) by Sharon Palmer, RD.

CHOCOLATE

Here's the skinny—chocolate is a sweet treat made from cacao beans, the fruit of the tropical *Theobroma cacao* tree. First, the cacao beans are fermented, dried, roasted and ground into cocoa liquor. The cocoa liquor is then separated into cocoa butter (a solid fat) and cocoa powder. These are combined with ingredients such as chocolate liquor (made by grinding the center of the cacao bean), sugar, milk or cream, and flavors to produce what some, including me, refer to as "the food of the gods."

Besides being a delicious addition to any diet, chocolate has come out of the dark in recent years, both literally and figuratively, owing to its potential to help our hearts stay healthy. Chocolate is rich in antioxidants. In fact, it's one of the most concentrated sources of polyphenol antioxidants called flavonoids. The 2006 and 2010 studies about antioxidant-rich herbs and spices described earlier (see page 127) showed chocolate to be a queen for its antioxidant properties. The 2006 study found unsweetened baking chocolate, dark chocolate and milk chocolate candy to be among the top fifty foods (out of 1,113) with the highest antioxidant content. The 2010 study also found chocolate to be rich in antioxidants. In both studies, the researchers found the average antioxidant content to be higher when the cocoa content was higher and the chocolate was less processed. Too much processing, for example, to make milk chocolate, destroys many beneficial antioxidant compounds. An article in *Alternative Therapies* in 2001 reported that after processing, milk chocolate is between 7 and 35 percent cacao, and dark chocolate is between 30 and 80 percent cacao. Dark chocolate also, typically, has roughly twice the antioxidants as milk chocolate. And sorry you milk chocolate fans, but studies also suggest that milk proteins found in milk chocolate inhibit flavonoid absorption.

Here's the bad news. Although the nutrient composition of chocolate varies depending on the kind you buy, most chocolate packs a high dose of calories, mainly from sugar and fat, especially saturated fat. Fortunately, about half the saturated fat found in chocolate is stearic acid, a kind of fat that has neutral effects on blood cholesterol levels. And the good news is chocolate contains some healthy fats, especially monounsaturated fatty acids, and key nutrients, including copper and phosphorus (see Vital Nutrients: Milk

Chocolate vs. Dark Chocolate). And for those of you who claim to get a chocolate high, chocolate also contains several stimulants, including caffeine and anandamide, a substance associated with a mild sense of euphoria.

Craving Chocolate? Let Your Nose Know!

A study published in *Appetite* in 2012 found that smelling jasmine significantly reduced chocolate cravings. And a study that appeared in *Addictive Behavior* in 2013 found that smelling a neutral, unfamiliar odorant reduced cravings for highly desired foods, including chocolate. Researchers believe that cravings and odors compete for limited resources, and that some odors are able to reduce cravings.

Vital Nutrients: Milk Chocolate vs. Dark Chocolate

Here's a side-by-side nutritional comparison of one ounce of dark chocolate and one ounce of milk chocolate.

Chocolate	Calories	Total Fat (g)	MUFA[a] (g)	PUFA[b] (g)	SFA[c] (g)	Other Vital Nutrients
Dark chocolate (70–85% cacao solids)	170	12.1	3.6	0.4	6.9	manganese[1] copper[1] iron[2] magnesium[2] phosphorus[3] zinc[3] potassium[3]
Milk chocolate	151	9.4	2	0.4	5.2	copper[3] manganese[3] phosphorus[3] calcium[3]

a Monounsaturated fatty acids; **b** Polyunsaturated fatty acids; **c** Saturated fatty acids.

1 Provides at least 20 percent of the Daily Value of the nutrient (an excellent source); **2** Provides 10 to 19 percent of the Daily Value of the nutrient (a good source); **3** Provides 5 to less than 10 percent of the Daily Value of the nutrient.

Source: U.S. Department of Agriculture, Agricultural Research Service. 2012. USDA National Nutrient Database for Standard Reference, Release 25. Nutrient Data Laboratory Home Page, www.ars.usda.gov/nutrientdata.

HEALTH BENEFITS OF CHOCOLATE

More good news for chocoholics: over the last decade, countless studies have suggested that consuming polyphenol-rich cocoa and chocolate can protect your heart. A study published in *Clinical Nutrition* in 2011 found that consuming chocolate was inversely related to coronary heart disease. Several other studies have concluded that consuming cocoa or chocolate can benefit your heart and health by:

1. **Lowering blood pressure levels.** Consuming chocolate has been shown to lower blood pressure, at least over the short term. Although the mechanisms are unknown, some studies suggest that substances in chocolate called flavanols lower blood pressure. In a 2012 review of several short-term studies, Australian researchers found that consuming chocolate and cocoa products had a small but statistically significant effect in lowering blood pressure. A review published in *Archives of Internal Medicine* in 2007 determined that the consumption of cocoa-rich foods was correlated with reduced blood pressure levels. And in a study published in *Current Drug Delivery* in 2011, researchers found significantly lower blood pressure levels in adults who reported higher dark chocolate consumption than in those who ate less dark chocolate. Also, increasing dark chocolate intake was associated with a significant decrease in blood pressure values, regardless of age or family history of hypertension.

2. **Lowering cholesterol levels.** In a review published in the *European Journal of Clinical Nutrition* in 2011, researchers found that consuming dark chocolate and cocoa products led to significant reductions in total cholestrol and LDL (bad) cholesterol levels.

3. **Lowering insulin levels.** A review published in the *American Journal of Clinical Nutrition* in 2012 concluded that consuming chocolate or cocoa led to significant reductions in insulin levels and, therefore, insulin resistance (a precursor to type 2 diabetes) among 1,297 participating.

4. **Making you feel good.** Eating chocolate may have a positive effect on your mood. In a randomized, double-blind study, researchers gave seventy-two healthy middle-aged adults a dark chocolate drink mix that provided varying

amounts of polyphenol antioxidants (the placebo had none) once daily for thirty days. The study, published in the *Journal of Psychopharmacology,* found that those who drank the drinks with the highest polyphenol dose rated themselves as significantly more calm and content than those who had the polyphenol-free drink. And in a two-week study published in *Nutrients* in 2012, researchers found that among 90 eighteen- to thirty-five-year-olds, those who had high anxiety levels reported feeling less anxiety after consuming milk chocolate within an hour following a meal.

Here's my bottom line: if you like chocolate, there's no reason why you shouldn't have it in small quantities or as an occasional splurge. In a review that appeared in *Antioxidants and Redox Signaling* in 2011, Yale University researchers concluded that the antioxidant and anti-inflammatory benefits of chocolate and cocoa, which promote heart health, reduce insulin resistance, reduce inflammation and provide cognitive and mood benefits, outweigh any negatives associated with their consumption. So have some chocolate if you wish. Just be sure to limit yourself to small portions and eat only the kinds you love. I explain how to fit the extra calories in chocolate into your Vitality Diet in Chapter 12.

Vital R$_x$

Antioxidants

- Eat your fruits and vegetables daily, ideally including some with each meal and snack. Options that provide an excellent source of vitamin C, a key antioxidant nutrient, include berries, citrus fruits, cantaloupe, artichokes, asparagus, Brussels sprouts, kale, spinach and tomatoes.
- To flavor foods, swap some (or all) of the salt you use while you prepare, cook or eat food for herbs and spices, especially dried versions.
- Treat yourself with small amounts of dark chocolate or even milk chocolate. To limit portions, have it right after meals instead of in between.

CHAPTER

9

DRINK CLEAN AND GET THE REAL DEAL ON CAFFEINE

Dehydration is a major vitality zapper. Did you know that being even slightly dehydrated can increase levels of cortisol? And that high levels of cortisol have been shown to speed up aging? Dehydration is also associated with weathered skin, brain drain and fatigue. Although it's hard to tell how close Americans come to meeting current fluid intake recommendations (see Water on page 139), a study in the *Journal of the American Dietetic Association* in 1999 estimated that as many as two-thirds of us are somewhat dehydrated at any given time. And if you're already feeling stressed and overwhelmed to begin with, fluid loss as little as 1 or 2 percent of your body weight (that's one to two pounds of fluid for every one hundred pounds you weigh) can take its toll on your physical and emotional health, as shown in a study published in the *Journal of Nutrition* in 2012. Twenty-five young women who had moderate exercise-induced dehydration that led to a fluid loss of 1.36 percent of their body weight experienced dampened mood, a lowered ability to concentrate, headache and other symptoms.

Some of us may not hydrate enough, and that becomes a problem particularly when the seasons change and we sweat less and when we get older and our thirst sensation slips a little (see Vitality Check: Are You Drinking Enough? on page 137). But others are drinking too much of the wrong thing. And by that I mean they are drinking too many high-calorie, nutrient-poor beverages, including sugary soda, sweetened coffee concoctions, sports or energy drinks, and alcoholic beverages.

Do You Need to Cut Back on the Bubbly?

When you're stressed, it's hard to see things clearly. And if you drink alcoholic beverages to cope, you may even have a tougher time realizing when you're on the verge of having, or actually have, a problem. If you choose to drink alcohol, having no more than one drink a day or up to seven per week, as encouraged by current Dietary Guidelines for Americans, will reduce your chances of having problems in the future. But if you currently drink more than that, here are some Stressipes to help you cut back:

1. **Stressipe: Press Pause.** In her book *Sober for Good,* Anne Fletcher recommends that people pause and make a list of the current problems in their lives and then ask themselves, "Is alcohol connected to any of them? Is my drinking a common denominator in my troubles? Could I handle my problems better if it weren't for the way I use alcohol?"

2. **Stressipe: Be Smart When You're Social.** To cut back on social drinking, Fletcher recommends having a snack before heading to any event to prevent yourself from running on empty and to minimize alcohol's physiological effects. When you're at the event or venue, stand or linger far from the bar or cocktail table to reduce temptation. She also suggests alternating alcoholic beverages with nonalcoholic ones and/or keeping a glass of water or seltzer on hand to alternate sips.

3. **Stressipe: Create New Habits.** If you have certain habits that you pair with drinking, such as coming home from work and having a few glasses of wine, Fletcher suggests creating new habits—for instance, taking a walk with someone special to unwind at the end of your day. Similarly, if you have specific gal (or guy) pals that you drink with, suggest a new venue (the gym or the park) or an activity (a fitness or art class) to spend time together without the temptation to drink.

While small amounts of alcoholic drinks can be part of your Vitality Diet (I explain how in Chapter 12), they don't provide the key nutrients we need to achieve the 7 Pillars of Vitality. Although estimates vary, on average we Americans drink about twenty out of every one hundred calories we consume. That means that sugary sodas, sports and energy drinks, caloric sweetened coffee beverages and even alcoholic beverages take up about one-fifth of our daily energy intake.

Stressipe

Redefine Your Nightcap.

When you eat out–at a restaurant or at a party or another event–make a decision beforehand about what and how much you'll eat or drink based on what you've already eaten that day. Curb your calorie load by ordering one or two appetizers, including healthfully prepared vegetables, instead of a full entrée, and by having up to one drink (if you must). Otherwise, drink a low-calorie beverage, such as sparkling water with a splash of 100 percent fruit juice. When you've had enough–even if you haven't eaten everything–cap off your meal by putting on some lipstick or popping in a breath strip, a strong mint or chewing gum.

Although some of those beverages do supply valuable nutrients and can count toward meeting your hydration needs, many simply contain lots of calories and added sugars that we just don't need.

Vitality Check ✓

Are You Drinking Enough?

Lawrence E. Armstrong, PhD, of the University of Connecticut, Human Performance Laboratory, offers three suggestions to tell if you're dehydrated:

1. **Use your weight.** Armstrong recommends weighing yourself on three consecutive days to determine your baseline body weight. Losing one pound may indicate mild dehydration. Armstrong recommends using the expression "A pint's a pound the world around" as a reminder that if your weight goes down by a pound, you should replace the lost fluid by drinking one pint (two cups) of water.

continued on page 138

2. **Assess the color.*** According to Armstrong, if your urine has a deep hue and is not "pale yellow" or "straw colored," you may also need more fluid (although some medications and dietary supplements can affect the color of urine).

3. **Let thirst be your guide.** Although Armstrong says thirst is often criticized as an inadequate marker for hydration, he says that if you feel thirsty—especially between bedtime and morning—you're probably mildly dehydrated. Armstrong says, "If you notice one out of three signs—for example, your urine has a deep color—it is likely that you're mildly dehydrated. If you have two out of the three signs—you've lost at least one pound and you feel thirsty—it's very likely you're mildly dehydrated.

*Visit www.hydrationcheck.com to obtain more information and to order a color chart to assess the color of your urine.

Although incorporating a wide variety of nutrient-rich Vital Foods is encouraged when following the Vitality Diet, when it comes to Vital Drinks, I say, "Keep it simple." When choosing your beverages, think first about which drinks will give you the most in terms of hydration. Building adequate hydration into your day can give you a vitality boost and help:

- Maintain your skin's moisture.

- Increase your mental performance.

- Boost your mood—even slight dehydration can leave you feeling irritable and cranky.

- Quell hunger pangs—the hunger and thirst mechanisms are located near each other in the brain, so sometimes when you think you feel hungry, you may actually be thirsty.

Besides thinking about hydration, it's important to consider which drinks are most likely to supply your body and brain with key nutrients and also lift you up when you rise in the morning, energize you daily and settle you down when you're trying to sleep. Read on to learn more about the Vital Drinks—water, tea, milk and 100 percent fruit juice.

WATER

Water is arguably the most critical component of your Vitality Diet. That's because while we can go for weeks without food, we literally can't survive without water for more than a few days. More than half of our body weight is water, which plays a key role. It:

- Carries oxygen and nutrients to muscles and helps eliminate wastes, such as carbon dioxide and lactic acid, from your body.

- Regulates body temperature, prevents dehydration and reduces fluid retention, which can strain your heart.

- Moisturizes your skin, ears, nose and throat and protects joints, organs and body tissues from injury.

- Supports healthy digestion by being a key component of saliva and gastric juices and by helping fiber pass through your body.

The Institute of Medicine of the National Academy of Sciences recommends a total of eleven and a half cups (2.7 liters) of water daily for women aged nineteen and older. Of that, about two and a half cups can come from produce and cooked grains. Women who are physically active or athletic, who live in or spend time in warm climates or at high altitudes, and who have medical conditions that contribute to fluid retention have higher water needs.

WHY IT'S GOOD TO HAVE WATER WEIGHT

While some studies suggest that consuming water from foods, such as fruits, vegetables, soups and cooked grains, like oatmeal, is associated with a lower body mass index (BMI) and a smaller waist circumference, other studies suggest that water intake at breakfast and lunch can reduce energy or calorie consumption. In a study published in the *Journal of the American Dietetic Association* in 2008, researchers gave twenty-four overweight and obese older men and women a standard breakfast on two separate occasions. Thirty minutes before the meal, some subjects were given a little more than two cups of water and some were not. The researchers found that those who drank water before the meal had a significantly lower calorie intake (13 percent) than those who did not. In another study, this one published in *Obesity* in 2007, researchers gave non-obese younger and older subjects about one and a half cups of water thirty minutes before a standard lunch on one occasion, and no water on another occasion. Although the younger subjects' energy intake at lunch was not significantly different whether they drank the water or not, older subjects consumed significantly fewer calories when they drank water before the meal compared with when they did not.

And if you're trying to lose weight, drinking more water may help you be even more successful. In a twelve-week study published in *Obesity* in 2010, researchers assigned forty-eight overweight or obese middle-aged or older adults either to a reduced-calorie diet with about two cups of water before each meal or to the reduced-calorie diet without the water. At the start of the study and then at twelve weeks, each subject had two test meals, one served without water and one served with the water (about two cups) thirty minutes before the meal. The researchers found that those who consumed water before meals lost 44 percent more weight—about 4.4 pounds—than those who did not.

Although more data is needed to determine the relationship between water and body weight, staying hydrated is reason enough for you to give water the weight it deserves.

Do It or Ditch It?

Bottled Water

According to the Beverage Marketing Corporation, bottled water sales have boomed in recent years. It found that a record-high 9.7 billion gallons (30.8 gallons per person) of bottled water was sold in the United States in 2012 alone. But consider this: while drinking a lot of bottled water, especially the unsweetened, plain kind, can help you hydrate, all that leftover plastic harms the environment. According to Kate Geagan, MS, RD, America's Green Nutritionist and the author of *Go Green, Get Lean*, "Disposable plastic bottles are mostly petroleum based; in fact, about 17 million barrels of oil a year are used to make and ship them." She adds, "People also pay up to 5,000 times more for bottled water than tap (imagine paying 5,000 times more for a sandwich or anything else in your diet). Bottled water is also two to four times as expensive as gasoline." Geagan also says that it often takes more water to manufacture a plastic water bottle than the amount you'll find in the bottle. Because tap water is also more tightly regulated than bottled water, Geagan recommends replacing plastic water bottles with environmentally friendly reusable ones that are free of bisphenol A (BPA)—a chemical used to make plastic that has been linked with adverse health effects in animal studies—to minimize the footprint left by your hydration habits.

SELTZER, CLUB SODA AND TONIC WATER

Although carbonated waters can be a part of your overall fluid intake, they're often acidic and can contribute to dental erosion. Flavored store-bought varieties, as well as your own concoctions made with a splash of 100 percent fruit juice or fresh lemon, lime or orange slices, also can be acidic. Besides their corrosive effects on your teeth, carbonated waters can be significant sources of sodium, especially if you drink several daily or each week (read labels, since sodium amounts can vary considerably). For example, one cup of club soda has fifty milligrams of sodium, versus nine milligrams in one cup of tap water. And unlike naturally calorie-free tap water, seltzer and club soda, one cup of tonic water has a whopping eighty-three calories. So while it's better for your dental health and overall health to consume plain rather than fizzy waters, seltzer, club soda and similar carbonated waters that are calorie-free by definition can be part of your Vitality Diet. Just rinse with water soon after drinking them to help minimize damage to your tooth enamel. And if you can't live without a gin and tonic or other tonic cocktails, be sure to count those calories as Treats (see Chapter 12).

Vitality Check ✓

Should You Use Artificial Sweeteners and Sugar Substitutes?

Nothing is as much of a hot-button issue as artificial sweeteners and their place, if any, in a healthy diet. These sweeteners (found in pink, yellow and blue packets) are also ingredients in diet drinks, including sodas, teas, fruit drinks, and vitamin waters, and sugar-free products, including chewing gum, mints and candies, snacks, and desserts. Despite limited emerging research that suggests that sugar substitutes increase the appetite by causing calorie disregulation (disrupting the body's natural ability to determine which foods and beverages have calories and which don't based on the their taste and texture), a review of several studies by the Academy of Nutrition and Dietetics concluded that consuming artificial sweeteners does not increase appetite, hunger sensation or food intake in adults, nor does consuming them necessarily result in a less healthful diet. The Academy also determined, based on limited research on humans, that artificial sweeteners (see FDA-Approved Sugar Substitutes on page 142) are safe for use in most people. (Pregnant women, however, are advised to avoid saccharin and to use only FDA-approved sugar substitutes in moderate amounts, and individuals with phenylketonuria

continued on page 142

[PKU], a rare genetic disorder, should avoid aspartame because it contains phenylalanine, which their bodies cannot break down.) Despite this conclusion, the Centers for Science in the Public Interest, an independent science-based organization, urges Americans to avoid FDA-approved additives,* including saccharin, aspartame and acesulfame-K, because they're unsafe in the amounts consumed or are poorly tested and not worth any risk. My recommendation is to play it safe and to limit or avoid artificially sweetened foods and beverages. Instead, get your fix from naturally sweet foods like fruit and limited amounts of 100 percent fruit juice.

*For more on food additives, visit www.cspinet.org/reports/chemcuisine.htm#safety_summary.

FDA-Approved Sugar Substitutes

The following six sweeteners are approved for use by the U.S. Food and Drug Administration (FDA). (Any mention of brand-name items should not be construed as an implied endorsement.):

Acesulfame-K *(Sunett)*

Aspartame *(Equal, NutraSweet)*

Neotame (not currently available for consumer purchase)

Saccharin *(Sweet'N Low)*

Stevia/Rebiana *(Truvia, Pure Via)*

Sucralose *(Splenda)*

TEA

Drinking tea is linked with many vital health benefits, which are attributed to tea's high amount of polyphenols (specifically flavonoids), powerful plant chemicals that not only act as antioxidants to fight free-radical damage but also have anti-inflammatory and antiviral benefits. Studies suggest that sipping tea can protect your heart, your skin and your bones. Tea also may help you manage stress, may support healthy cognition, may aid in weight management and may even protect against cancer and type 2 diabetes.

TEA AND YOUR HEART

Some studies suggest that drinking tea—green, black, white and even herbal teas—may reduce the risk of cardiovascular disease, including stroke, and may reduce the risk of death from cardiovascular disease and other causes. These benefits are likely because of tea's potent mix of polyphenols. Here are some recent findings:

- According to a clinical trial published in *Preventive Medicine* in 2012, drinking a little less than one cup of black tea three times a day led to significant decreases in fasting serum glucose (raised levels increase type 2 diabetes risk) and improvements in blood lipids, including triglycerides, HDL (good) cholesterol, and LDL (bad) cholesterol (reducing cardiovascular risk). Researchers also found an increase in subjects' overall antioxidant status.

- In a study that appeared in *Arteriosclerosis, Thrombosis and Vascular Biology* in 2010, researchers found that drinking three to six cups of tea daily was associated with a 45 percent lower risk of death from coronary heart disease.

- In a review of seventeen studies, published in the *American Journal of Epidemiology* in 2001, researchers found that the risk of having a heart attack was reduced by 11 percent in those who increased their tea intake to three cups daily.

- In a review published in *Stroke* in 2009, researchers analyzed nine studies and found that drinking three cups of green or black tea daily was associated with a reduced risk of stroke.

TEA AND YOUR SKIN

A study that appeared in the *Journal of Nutrition* in 2011 found that drinking green tea improved women's overall skin quality and protected them against skin damage caused by UV radiation. As part of the study, subjects drank a green tea or placebo beverage. Their skin was assessed initially and again at six and twelve weeks. After being exposed to UV radiation, skin redness or inflammation was reduced by 16 percent at six weeks and 25 percent at twelve weeks in women who drank green tea. They also experienced improved skin elasticity and less roughness and scaling, and they had better blood flow and oxygen delivery to their skin.

TEA AND YOUR BONES

A study published in the *American Journal of Clinical Nutrition* in 2000 found that among sixty-five- to seventy-six-year-old women, those who drank tea had significantly greater mean bone mineral density measurements than those who did not. The researchers speculated that the effects are due to the bone-friendly flavonoids found in tea. They also suggested that tea drinking may protect against osteoporosis in older women. Several studies have also shown an association between higher tea intake and improved bone mineral density and a reduced fracture risk in older women.

TEA AND STRESS

In a study published in the *American Journal of Clinical Nutrition* in 2009, researchers found that among more than forty thousand adults aged forty and above, those who consumed at least five cups of green tea daily were 20 percent less likely to be stressed than those who had one cup daily. Although it's unclear why drinking green tea may have these effects, researchers speculate that theanine, an amino acid found in green tea, which acts like a natural relaxant, tranquilizing the brain without sedating, may play a role. Another study, this one published in *Psychopharmacology* in 2007, found that men who drank four cups of black tea daily for six weeks had lower cortisol levels and rated themselves as more relaxed than those who consumed a placebo beverage.

TEA AND YOUR BRAIN

According to a review in *Nutrition Reviews* in 2008, drinking caffeinated tea at regular intervals can help you maintain alertness, focused attention, and accuracy and may modulate the more acute effects of higher doses of caffeine.

Iced or Hot: Which Is Better?

In a study published in the *European Journal of Nutrition* in 2012, researchers looked at the link between the intake of hot or iced tea (either sweetened or unsweetened) and weight and other markers for metabolic syndrome, that cluster of conditions that includes high blood pressure and abdominal obesity, which increases the risk for cardiovascular disease and diabetes. In a nationally representative sample of almost sixty-five hundred adults, the researchers found that regular or daily consumers of hot tea had smaller waist sizes and lower body mass indexes compared with nondrinkers. Interestingly, iced tea drinkers had larger waist sizes and body mass indexes compared with nondrinkers. Hot tea intake, but not iced tea, was also associated with heart-health benefits, such as increased HDL (good) cholesterol levels and decreased levels of CRP (a marker for inflammation).

When asked about why hot tea drinkers seemed to fare better than iced tea drinkers, lead researcher Jaqueline Vernarelli, PhD, explained, "It's possible that individuals who drink iced tea have a different overall dietary pattern than those who drink hot tea—the iced tea may serve as a marker for dietary behavior. For example, if one person habitually drinks sweet tea and also eats barbecue ribs, they'd have a very different dietary profile than a person who habitually drinks hot tea and eats sushi. It is also possible that the iced tea may have a lower amount of phenolic compounds, and therefore not have the same metabolic effects as hot tea." She added, "Based on the data, we know that hot tea consumption is associated with a lower risk of obesity-related diseases in American adults."

Although a lot more data is needed, animal studies suggest that green tea may protect against different kinds of cancer, in large part because of the polyphenol antioxidants it provides.

COFFEE

Coffee is one of the most consumed beverages around the world. Whether they call it java or joe or just plain coffee, many count on coffee to wake up or stay alert and focused throughout the day. Made from ground beans, coffee contains more than a thousand compounds. These include:

- Chlorogenic acid, a major phenolic compound that acts as an antioxidant.

- Caffeine, a central nervous system stimulant that is rapidly absorbed and then dispersed to the brain and all body tissues (see Caffeine: A Shield for Your Skin? on page 146).

- Cafestol and kahweol, fat-soluble compounds known as diterpenes (espresso and other unfiltered coffee drinks contain high levels). While they have been shown to have anticancer and anti-inflammatory properties, they (especially cafestol) have also been shown to raise total cholesterol, LDL (bad) cholesterol and triglyceride levels.

Coffee also contains very small doses of some vitamins and minerals. Because it has a very high water content, coffee (like tea) can help you stay hydrated.

Caffeine: A Shield for Your Skin?

Did you know that consuming caffeine might be good for your skin? In a study published in *Cancer Research* in 2012, researchers determined that caffeine intake from all dietary sources (including tea, cola and chocolate) was inversely associated with the risk of basal cell carcinoma (BCC). Women who consumed more than three cups of caffeinated (not decaffeinated) coffee daily also had a significantly lower risk than those who consumed less than one cup per month. A previous study published in the *European Journal of Cancer Prevention* found that among Caucasian women, those who drank caffeinated coffee daily had a 10.8 percent lower prevalence of non-melanoma skin cancer. Researchers also found that consuming six or more cups of caffeinated (and not decaffeinated) coffee was associated with a 30 percent reduced prevalence of non-melanoma skin cancer. Although more studies are needed, researchers believe that caffeine protects the skin by killing off skin cells that become damaged by UV light.

COFFEE AND DISEASE

Countless studies have looked at the link between coffee and disease risk. According to a study published in *Missouri Medicine* in 2011, emerging research suggests that coffee intake is correlated with a lower risk of type 2 diabetes, stroke, depression, death from any cause, and Alzheimer's and other neurodegenerative diseases. In another review, this one published in *Critical Reviews in Food Science Nutrition* in 2011, researchers noted that, besides the many studies that illustrate that increased coffee intake is associated with a reduced risk of type 2 diabetes, several types of cancer, and neurodegenerative diseases (like Alzheimer's disease), consuming coffee has also been shown to reduce oxidative stress (thereby inhibiting aging) and improve cognitive function. A previous review in the same journal in 2006 concluded that, despite its potential disease-reducing benefits, drinking coffee may boost blood pressure and homocysteine levels—both risk factors for cardiovascular disease.

Do It or Ditch It?

Caffeine

For many of us, caffeine seems to offer some perks. If you're short on sleep, having some coffee or tea can truly feel like the best part of waking up. That's because caffeine binds to adenosine receptors in the brain to prevent the adenosine, a part of our genetic material, from acting as a natural relaxant. But numerous studies suggest that many of the cognitive or neurological perks may be dampened when you use caffeine regularly since your body develops a tolerance to its effects. Although most experts suggest that up to three hundred or four hundred milligrams of caffeine (the amount you'd find in three to four cups of brewed coffee, six to eight cups of brewed black tea, or six to eight cans of caffeinated sodas—not the amped-up kinds) daily may actually benefit health, you may want to curb or forgo caffeine if any of the following apply to you:

- You get restless, shaky or anxious or feel your heart beat faster when you consume caffeine.
- You're at risk for or have hypertension.
- You're prone to stress.
- You have sleep problems.
- You're prone to headaches.
- You have acid reflux or a stomach ulcer.
- Your breasts are lumpy and painful.

If you decide you overdo caffeine and want to cut back, or if you need to cut back on caffeine or eliminate it completely for medical or other reasons, see How to Curb Caffeine on page 148.

Coffee intake has also been shown to protect against death. A large prospective study published in the *New England Journal of Medicine* in 2012 found that, among more than four hundred thousand men and women, drinking coffee was inversely associated with death from all causes, as well as death caused by heart disease, respiratory disease, stroke, injuries and accidents, diabetes, and infections.

How to Curb Caffeine Intake

If you know that you rely too heavily or are too dependent on caffeinated sodas, iced tea, energy drinks or coffee drinks to give you a lift, it's time to curb it or cut it—particularly if your caffeine intake interferes with your sleep or makes you jittery or anxious when you have it or go without it when you're used to having it. Although there's no current recommended intake for caffeine, most experts urge a maximum of three hundred to four hundred milligrams daily for most healthy people. Here are some Stressipes to help you cut back on your caffeine intake painlessly:

1. **Stressipe: Pace yourself.** Before you reduce your caffeine intake, keep a log of everything you consume that has caffeine in it (including chocolate and medications) for several days, and note when you have them. Going cold turkey can trigger fatigue and rebound headaches. Instead, set a goal to gradually reduce your intake by decreasing portion sizes (order the twelve-ounce cup of coffee instead of your usual twenty-ounce cup) or reducing the frequency with which you consume caffeine.

2. **Stressipe: Plan your fix.** If you don't want to give up caffeine altogether, decide the time of day that's most important for you to get your fix. If you rely on that morning cup of coffee to wake you up or as something you enjoy with a friend or spouse, have it then.

3. **Stressipe: Drink by day.** Try to limit your caffeine intake to only morning and early afternoon. Drinking caffeinated beverages too long after lunchtime might interfere with your ability to fall asleep at bedtime and stay asleep. That's because it may take up to half of a twenty-four-hour day for caffeine to completely clear your bloodstream. Drinking it before you hit the sheets may also cause you to wake up overnight to make a bathroom run.

4. **Stressipe: Find alternatives.** To curb caffeine, you can swap caffeinated coffee or tea for decaffeinated varieties. You may need to experiment to find a brand you enjoy. To get the fizz of soda, replace diet or sugary soda with sparkling water with lemon, lime or orange sections or other fresh fruit, or a splash of 100 percent fruit juice. If you usually drink diet soda, diet iced tea or other caffeinated, calorie-free beverages, be mindful not to replace them with high-calorie, nutrient-poor drinks—especially if you don't cut calories elsewhere.

Soda, Coffee and Depression

In a study presented at the American Academy of Neurology's annual meeting in San Diego, California, in March 2013, researchers from the National Institutes of Health looked at the link between the intake of soda, including diet soda, coffee and fruit drinks, and depression risk. Almost two hundred sixty-four thousand adults between the ages of fifty and seventy-one answered questions about their usual beverage consumption between 1995 and 1996. From 2004 to 2006, those same adults were asked if they were diagnosed with depression anytime since the year 2000. Researchers found that adults who regularly consumed four or more cans of soda or fruit punch daily were 30 percent more likely to have been diagnosed with depression than people who did not drink soda. Those who drank four cans of fruit punch daily were 38 percent more likely to have been diagnosed with depression than those who did not. Coffee drinkers fared far better: those who drank at least four cups daily were 10 percent less likely than non-coffee drinkers to have been diagnosed with depression. Although this study doesn't prove that drinking diet soda increases depression risk, or that drinking coffee prevents it, it suggests that cutting back on sugar-sweetened or artificially sweetened beverages or drinking coffee may help protect against depression.

MILK

Full disclosure: I drink milk every day and feed it to my children. I was even a spokesperson for the Got Milk campaign a few years ago, and I have done some talks on behalf of the dairy industry. I enjoy milk in my cereal or on its own, and I drink chocolate milk, either when I wake up or after a workout. (There's evidence that chocolate milk is a great post-exercise recovery beverage.) One cup of nonfat milk not only packs a one-two punch of both calcium and vitamin D, but it is also an excellent source of iodine, riboflavin and phosphorus and a good source of potassium, selenium and vitamin A.

VITAL PERKS OF MILK

Milk not only helps your bones stay strong, mainly because of the calcium, magnesium, phosphorous, vitamin D and protein it provides, but it also seems to protect your teeth and helps them stay pearly. Casein, a protein in milk, creates a thin film on your teeth that protects enamel from erosion from acidic foods and beverages and protects against cavities. A 2013 study published in the *Journal of the American Dental Association* found that drinking milk after eating sugary cereal reduced plaque acid levels that could erode tooth enamel and contribute to cavities. There's also evidence that drinking milk reduces disease risk. A review published in *Lipids* in 2010 found that adults with the highest milk and dairy intake had lower risks of all-cause death, heart disease, stroke and diabetes compared with adults who consumed the lowest amounts.

Drinking milk and eating dairy products may also play a role in weight management. Studies suggest that those who include dairy products, including milk, in their diet have a lower body weight than those who do not. A 2009 review in *Physician and Sports Medicine* also suggests that components of milk and dairy foods, including calcium and whey protein, may protect against the development of obesity.

Vitality Check ✓

What If I Don't Drink Milk?

You don't *need* to drink milk to follow the Vitality Diet, though I recommend it. But even if you have lactose intolerance, you may be able to tolerate small amounts of milk (for example, half a cup with meals). Flavored milks, like low-fat chocolate milk, may be better tolerated than plain white milk. You can also buy lactose-free milk or take chewable enzymes, like Lactaid. (Before taking these, be sure to discuss the matter with a doctor or a registered dietitian, especially if you take medications or use herbal or other dietary supplements.) And if you don't drink milk or eat yogurt or cheese, be sure to get much-needed calcium from beans and other calcium-rich foods (see Chapter 7). Also note that other than fortified soy beverages, many milk alternatives are not equal replacements for cow's milk in terms of nutrients (see Milks [Minus the Cow] on page 152).

Milks (Minus the Cow)*

Here are some vital stats for 1 cup (8 fluid ounces) of some of your favorite non-dairy milks. (Any mention of brand-name items should not be construed as an implied endorsement.)

Milks	Calories	Total Fat (g)	SFA[1] (g)	MUFA[2] (g)	PUFA[3] (g)	Sodium (mg)	Cho[4] (g)	Fiber (g)	Sugars (g)	Pro[5](g)	Vital Nutrients*
Almond milk (Silk, original)	60	2.5	0	1.5	0.5	160	8	<1	7	1	Excellent source of calcium, vitamin D, riboflavin, vitamin E and vitamin B_{12}; Good source of vitamin A
Coconut milk (Silk, Pure Coconut, original)	80	5	5	0	0	45	7	0	6	1	Excellent source of calcium, vitamin D and vitamin B_{12}; Good source of vitamin A
Hemp milk (Tempt, original)	100	6	0.5	1	4.5	110	9	0	6	2	Excellent source of calcium, vitamin D, riboflavin, vitamin B_{12} and phosphorus; Good source of vitamin A and magnesium
Rice Dream (enriched, original)	120	2.5	0	1.5	0.5	100	23	0	10	1	Excellent source of calcium, vitamin D and vitamin B_{12}; Good source of vitamin A and phosphorus
Flax milk (Flax USA, original)	50	2.5	0	0	1.5	80	7	0	7	0	Excellent source of calcium, vitamin D and vitamin B_{12}; Good source of phosphorus and vitamin A
Oat milk (organic oat, original	130	2.5	0	0.7	0.8	115	24	2	19	4	Excellent source of calcium, vitamin D and riboflavin; Good source of vitamin A and iron

1 Saturated fatty acids; **2** Monounsaturated fatty acids; **3** Polyunsaturated fatty acids; **4** Carbohydrate; **5** Protein

continued on page 152

*Based on Daily Value. An excellent source provides at least 20 percent of the Daily Value of the nutrient; a good source provides 10 to 19 percent of the Daily Value of the nutrient.

Sources: U.S. Department of Agriculture, Agricultural Research Service. 2012. USDA National Nutrient Database for Standard Reference, Release 25. Nutrient Data Laboratory Home Page,
www.ars.usda.gov/nutrientdata
www.silk.com/products/original-almondmilk
www.silk.com/products/original-coconutmilk
www.livingharvest.com/products/nutrition-facts#milk
www.tastethedream.com/products/product/1467/202.php
www.flaxusa.com/products.php?page=flaxmilk
www.pacificfoods.com/food/non-dairy-beverages/nut-grain-beverages/organic-oat-original

JUICE

Not only are 100 percent fruit juices, such as orange, cranberry and grape, packed with natural sweetness, but they also boast Vital Nutrients. For example, 100 percent fruit juices tend to be excellent sources of vitamin C. One cup of orange juice even has a whopping 207 percent of the Daily Value of vitamin C (see Spotlight on OJ on page 153). Here are some of the star nutrients you'll find in some of your favorite 100 percent fruit juices:

- Orange juice is a good source of folate, thiamine and potassium and an excellent source of vitamin C.

- Grape juice (purple or white) is an excellent source of vitamin C and manganese.

- Cranberry juice is a good source of vitamin K and vitamin E and an excellent source of vitamin C.

- Apple juice is an excellent source of vitamin C.

- White grapefruit juice is a good source of potassium and an excellent source of vitamin C.

Despite the perks of juice, you may avoid 100 percent fruit juices, thinking that they cause weight gain or type 2 diabetes. Although drinking too much juice can contribute to excess calorie consumption, especially because it lacks fiber and isn't as filling as whole fruit, its impact on body weight and disease risk is unclear. Current Dietary Guidelines for Americans suggest that while 100 percent fruit juice can be part of a healthful diet, most fruit servings should be whole fruit—including fresh, canned and frozen varieties, as well as dried fruit with no sugar added—rather than juice. If you drink 100 percent fruit juice, be prudent and keep your servings to no more than half a cup to one cup to leave room for whole fruit in your diet.

Spotlight on OJ

In a 2012 study of more than eighty-eight hundred adults published in *Nutrition Journal,* researchers found that a higher percentage of regular orange juice drinkers met recommended intake levels for vitamin A, vitamin C, folate and magnesium than those who passed on the juice. Juice drinkers were also more likely to meet recommended intake levels for potassium, a "nutrient of concern" (see Chapter 7), and had higher intakes of whole fruit and whole grains. Orange juice drinkers also had a lower average body mass index and lower total cholesterol and LDL (bad) cholesterol levels and were 21 percent less likely to be obese.

Vital R$_x$

Drink Clean

- Aim for eight to nine cups of fluids (including water, club soda, seltzer, tea, coffee, cow's milk or fortified soy beverages and 100 percent fruit juices) daily. Drink more when you sweat a lot from exercise and/or hot weather.
- If you drink caffeinated beverages, such as coffee, tea or soda, have them early in the day (before 2:00 p.m.). Their consumption later in the day may interfere with your sleep.
- If you don't drink cow's milk or fortified soy beverages, be sure to get calcium from other sources, including cheese, yogurt, non-dairy milk beverages (preferably unsweetened varieties), leafy green vegetables and beans (see Calcium-Rich Foods on page 110).
- Limit 100 percent fruit juices to no more than one cup daily to leave room in your diet for fiber-rich fruit.

VITAL MOVES

Food isn't the only thing that affects your vitality. Did you know that physical activity is the ultimate antiaging remedy? Decades of research have proven that being active and engaging in regular, consistent exercise support each and every one of the 7 Pillars of Vitality. Emerging research also suggests that while working out at a gym, taking a dance class, doing yoga or going for a run can certainly provide you with plenty of physical, mental and health benefits, sitting less and being more active is equally, if not more, important when it comes to achieving and preserving vitality. In the pages that follow, you'll learn about how being physically active can work its magic to help you look and feel younger.

EXERCISE IMPROVES YOUR APPEARANCE

Regular exercise increases blood flow, which not only cools you off but also nourishes your skin with oxygen and nutrients, giving you a healthy glow. Exercise also boosts collagen production, which helps skin look supple, and supports healthy skin, naturally plumping it up to help it stay strong. Resistance exercise also contributes to building and preserving lean muscle mass and reducing fat, which helps improve the appearance of your skin and entire body. And, of course, exercise—especially the weight-bearing kind, like walking, dancing or weight training—can benefit your bones. A review published in the *International Journal of Endocrinology* in 2013 found that exercise led to statistically significant increases in measures of bone mineral density (BMD) in premenopausal women.

EXERCISE BOOSTS YOUR PHYSICAL, MENTAL AND SEXUAL ENERGY

You may think that exercising makes you tired. There's a lot of evidence that says otherwise. For example, a study by University of Georgia researchers published in *Psychotherapy and Psychosomatics* in 2008 found that sedentary people who complained of fatigue increased their energy levels by 20 percent and decreased fatigue by 65 percent after engaging in low-intensity exercise three times a week for just six weeks.

Exercise can also help improve cognitive performance. Several studies suggest that those who are fit perform better on cognitive tests than those who are not. Women who exercise also preserve their cognitive function better as they get older than their less fit sisters and friends.

And here's a juicy fact to motivate you even further! Exercise can also help you have more fun in bed. Don't believe me? A study published in the *Journal of Women's Health* in 2010 found that women who reported they exercised more during the menopausal transition and early postmenopause had greater sexual desire than those who exercised less or not at all. Exercise contributes to this deliciously beneficial effect by increasing blood flow and thereby boosting libido. Studies also suggest that exercise may boost arousal by activating the sympathetic nervous system—the part of the autonomic nervous system that helps regulate control of most internal organs and mediates the "fight or flight" stress response. And let's not forget that because exercise helps you look and feel better, you'll have that much more confidence when you're between the sheets.

EXERCISE HELPS YOU KEEP CALM AND CARRY ON

Studies suggest that exercise can enhance mood and act as a buffer against stress, anxiety and even depression. According to a review published in the *Scandinavian Journal of Public Health* in 2009, there is an inverse association between physical activity and stress. A previous study that appeared in the same journal found that increased leisure-time physical activity reduced adults' perceptions of a high level of stress and decreased life dissatisfaction. While researchers are still trying to determine why, studies speculate that regular exercise increases levels of tryptophan, an amino acid that crosses the blood-brain barrier to produce the "feel good," mood-boosting neurotransmitter serotonin. Exercise also pumps up the production of brain-derived neurotrophic factor (BDNF), a protein found in the brain (and other body tissues) that acts like an antiaging wonder drug to support neuronal health. Studies suggest that exercise—especially the vigorous kind—may lengthen telomeres, the protective caps on chromosomes, which may be shortened due to psychological distress or poor nutrition, thus helping to prevent or decrease cellular aging (see Stress, Exercise and Telomeres on page 157).

Aimee Crant-Oksa, aged forty-three, from Matawan, New Jersey, knows firsthand that becoming a regular exerciser can be a lifesaver. Having a heart-wrenching miscarriage and seeing her mother have a bad fall inspired her, an on-again, off-again exerciser, to get back on track once and for all. Having had these trying experiences made her realize how important it was for her to get back to caring for herself. She had always wanted to take up running but had never thought she could do it, that is, until she promised a friend she would do a 5K race. She says, "Competing in that race truly changed my life. When my mother got sick soon after that 5K, running saved me." Now, instead of eating—her usual go-to coping strategy—Aimee turns to exercise to clear her head and keep it together. She has since added swimming to her exercise regimen and so far has completed sprint, intermediate and olympic-distance triathalons. Being fit and active has become a way of life for Aimee, and she stays motivated by setting new fitness goals for herself. She's so proud of herself and knows she'll keep going—especially because she has a daughter, for whom she wants to model healthful habits.

According to some researchers, preserving or increasing the length of telomeres is associated with reducing stress. In a study published in *PLoS One* in 2010, researchers assessed perceived stress in sixty-three healthy postmenopausal women, dividing them into a sedentary group and an active group based on their reported vigorous physical activity. Researchers found that higher perceived stress was associated with shorter telomere length and that vigorous physical activity appeared to protect women who perceived high stress by acting as a buffer against shortened telomere length. Another study, this one published in the *American Journal of Epidemiology* in 2012, looked at activity level, sedentary behavior and telomere length in more than seventy-eight hundred women between the ages of forty-three and seventy and concluded that moderate activity may be associated with greater telomere length.

EXERCISE HELPS YOU MANAGE YOUR WEIGHT

Being physically active regularly may help you maintain your weight and may prevent excess weight gain. If you also cut calories, exercise can help contribute to weight loss and help you maintain your optimal weight in the long term. In fact, about 90 percent of successful long-term weight loss maintainers who are part of the National Weight Control Registry (NWCR)—the largest study of long-term weight loss behavior in adults, initiated by Rena Wing, PhD, and James O. Hill, PhD—report they exercise on average about an hour a day (mostly walking). Although most kinds of exercise can help your body burn calories, resistance exercise is especially effective at helping you build or preserve muscle, which keeps your metabolism working at high speed. A study published in *Obesity* in 2012 showed that NWCR subjects spent significantly more time doing moderate or vigorous physical activity than overweight subjects and marginally more than normal weight subjects. The researchers suggested that their results confirm how important physical activity, in bursts of at least ten minutes at a time, is to maintaining weight loss over the long term.

There's also evidence that exercise—even a short, brisk walk, which can easily be slipped into your day—can help you fight food cravings, which could contribute to excess calorie intake and subsequent weight gain. In a study published in *Medicine and Science in Sports and Exercise* in 2012, researchers measured brain waves in thirty-five women exposed to food images following a morning in which the women took a brisk forty-five-minute walk and one in which they did not. Researchers discovered that exercise dampened the arousal to food cues in the women who exercised, making them less likely to eat. In another study, one published in *Appetite* in 2012, researchers had seventy-eight regular chocolate consumers abstain from chocolate for two days. Subjects were then randomly asked to take a brisk fifteen-minute walk or enjoy quiet rest, followed by low- or high-demand tasks done at a desk (to simulate a work environment). A bowl of chocolates was available for them to consume at will. Researchers found that those who exercised before the tasks consumed half as much chocolate as those who did not exercise.

So many of the women I've worked with have struggled with finding the time to get fit. Consider Yvette Rivera, forty-two, a mother of two from New York City. After she turned forty, she began to put on weight and joined a gym. But getting there after work became more of a chore over time and she slacked off. One day she decided to try to exercise at work during her lunch hour. She began to walk the halls of her office building and take the stairs up and down five flights for forty-five minutes at least four days a week. In no time, she inspired colleagues to join her. She says, "Staying committed to exercise has always been a challenge, but doing it this way seems to work for me." Instead of lying on the couch after a hard day's work, Yvette now goes home and does some exercise with her fourteen-year-old son, Baby J. "My son is a great trainer who pushes and encourages me," she says. She adds, "Being fit helps me look and feel better than ever." The moral of the story? Where there's a will there's a way, and like Yvette, you, too, can find a way to fit in fitness and even make it a way to connect and spend quality time with others—and look and feel your best.

EXERCISE HELPS YOU GET YOUR Z'S

In a review of the effects of exercise on sleep published in *Frontiers in Neurology* in 2012, chronic exercise was shown to help you fall asleep faster and stay asleep longer. Exercise can also indirectly improve your shut-eye by having a beneficial effect on mood. In a review that appeared in the *Journal of Physiotherapy* in 2012, researchers noted that adults aged forty and older who participated in exercise training programs for ten and sixteen weeks had better sleep quality and fell asleep significantly faster than non-exercisers. Another study, this one published in the *British Medical Journal* in 2012, found that exercise—even in low doses—significantly improved sleep quality and reduced the odds of sleep disturbance in obese or overweight postmenopausal women. A review published in *Clinics (São Paulo)* in 2012 also concluded that exercise has been shown to reduce sleep problems and can effectively treat chronic insomnia. (See Chapter 11 for more about sleep.)

EXERCISE REDUCES DISEASE RISK

There are mountains of evidence to show that exercise boosts immune function, helping you fight off colds and flu, and has anti-inflammatory effects, helping you ward off serious health conditions, such as heart disease, diabetes, cancer and high blood pressure. Here are just some recent findings:

1. In a 2011 review published in *Circulation*, researchers found that adults who reported that they engaged in two and a half hours weekly of moderate

leisure-time physical activity, such as walking (which is the minimum amount recommended according to current federal guidelines; see Vitality Check: How Much Exercise is Enough?), had a 14 percent lower risk of coronary heart disease (CHD) compared with adults who reported no leisure-time physical activity. Adults who engaged in five hours per week of moderate-intensity leisure-time physical activity had a 20 percent lower risk of CHD.

2. In a review that appeared in *Diabetes Care* in 2007, researchers determined that adults who exercised regularly had a 31 percent lower risk for developing type 2 diabetes than those who were sedentary. Similarly, those who walked briskly for at least two and a half hours weekly had a 30 percent lower risk of type 2 diabetes compared with those who did almost no walking. Researchers concluded that moderate exercise, such as brisk walking, can substantially reduce type 2 diabetes risk.

3. A study published in the *American Journal of Epidemiology* in 2012 suggests that physical activity may be particularly effective in lowering blood pressure among salt-sensitive individuals.

Vitality Check ✓

How Much Exercise is Enough?

In 2008 the U.S. Department of Health and Human Services (HHS) issued science-based Physical Activity Guidelines for adults and children. For adults aged nineteen to sixty-four without health or medical conditions that limit their mobility, the recommendations for achieving modest health benefits include:

*   A weekly total of 150 minutes (two and a half hours) of aerobic exercise, with intervals of at least 10 minutes of moderate-intensity[1] aerobic physical activity, or 75 minutes of vigorous-intensity[2] physical activity or an equivalent combination of moderate- and vigorous-intensity aerobic physical activity.

For women who want additional benefits, the Physical Activity Guidelines recommend:

*   A weekly total of at least 300 minutes (five hours) of moderate-intensity or 150 minutes of vigorous-intensity aerobic activity or an equivalent combination of moderate- and vigorous-intensity aerobic physical activity.

The guidelines also recommend muscle-strengthening activities[3] that involve all major muscle groups at least two days a week.

1 Moderate-intensity physical activity is aerobic activity that moderately raises heart rate and breathing (for example, a 5 to 6 on a scale from 1 to 10). Examples include brisk walking, dancing, swimming or biking on a level terrain.

2 Vigorous-intensity physical activity is aerobic activity that greatly increases heart rate and breathing (for example, a 7 to 8 on a scale from 1 to 10). Examples include jogging, playing singles tennis, swimming laps or biking on hills.

3 Muscle-strengthening activity is physical activity that increases skeletal muscle strength, power, endurance and mass. It includes strength or resistance training and muscular strength and endurance exercise.

Source: U.S. Department of Health and Human Services. 2008 Physical Activity Guidelines for Americans. Washington (DC): US Department of Health and Human Services; 2008. ODPHP Publication No. U0036. www.health.gov/paguidelines.

Despite the amazing benefits exercise provides, few of us meet the 2008 Physical Activity Guidelines. According to the 2012 report *Health, United States, 2010*, by the HHS, the Centers for Disease Control and Prevention (CDC) and the National Center for Health Statistics (NCHS), in 2010 fewer than half of all adults aged eighteen and older met current guidelines for aerobic physical activity. Less than one quarter of adults met the guidelines for muscle-strengthening physical activity. Only one in five adults met the guidelines for both types of exercise. On top of those dismal statistics, many women spend countless hours seated while working at their desks, commuting, watching their kids' ball games or dance recitals, or simply vegging out in front of the TV. Unfortunately, emerging research suggests that your chair or couch can be a death trap in disguise. In a study published in the *Archives of Internal Medicine* in 2012, researchers found that among two hundred twenty-two thousand Australian adults, prolonged sitting increased their risk of death from all causes, including cardiovascular disease. A 2012 study in the *British Journal of Sports Medicine* that followed more than sixty-six hundred older women for nine years also found that prolonged sitting increased the risk of all-cause mortality. (See How to Avoid the Sitting Disease on page 162).

How to Avoid the Sitting Disease

When asked why she was standing in the back of the room at a conference while the rest of us were seated at our tables, listening to a lecture, dietitian Robyn Flipse said, "I don't want to get the sitting disease!" We all know how vital being active is, but sitting too much—even if we also do formal exercise or are otherwise physically active—can increase disease and death risk. Here are four Stressipes to help you sidestep "the sitting disease":

1. **Stressipe: Take ten.** For every hour you sit, take ten minutes to stand, stretch, take a short walk or climb some stairs. Set an alarm as a reminder. If you know you'll be sitting for prolonged periods at a conference or event, sit in an aisle seat toward the side or the back of the room so you'll have an easy escape.

2. **Stressipe: Walk while you talk.** If you know you'll be on a long conference call, or you simply need some extra time to get advice from or console a friend, plan to walk (or at least pace) while you talk. Better yet, take or make the call while walking in the park or on a treadmill to kill two birds with one phone!

3. **Stressipe: Measure your moves.** Wearing a pedometer or a cute watch or device (like a Jawbone Up or a Fitbit) or using an app or tracking device built into your phone to track your steps or miles are great ways to stay accountable and set goals for yourself. Although accumulating ten thousand steps a day (the equivalent of five miles, which includes the steps you take while exercising) is a common recommendation many experts make to maintain fitness, set your own pace by tracking your typical daily or weekly distance. Increase your mileage just a bit every day until you reach a daily average of ten thousand steps—or whatever goal you set for yourself (see Activity Conversion Chart for Women in Appendix A).

4. **Stressipe: Slip it in.** Except for a medical condition that keeps you off your feet, there's simply no excuse to not get up and move. Even while traveling, you can walk through an airport instead of taking elevators, escalators or moving sidewalks. Instead of sitting idly while waiting to get on a plane, work in extra mileage by just walking around nearby gates. On a road trip? Make scheduled stops to step outside, stand, stretch and breathe in some much-needed fresh air.

Now that you know why it's crucial to not only do regular formal exercise but also reduce sitting time each day, you'll do it, right? But if you're like many women who start a fitness routine, only to stop because of a million and one excuses—fatigue, lack of energy, a busy schedule, a demanding job, lack of sleep, family demands and the list goes on—remember, you can literally squeeze in short bursts of activity over the course of the day that add up to improved health and fitness. You don't need to run a marathon or do an Ironman Triathlon. It's far more important, and effective, to get active in a way that's realistic for you to maintain your health and to minimize your risk for exercise-related injuries (see Vitality Check: No Need for Extremes).

Whether you're just getting started or you already exercise regularly but just want to "shake up" your workout, you're likely to find that a few of the Vital Moves discussed below (including 7 Moves You Can't Refuse on page 167) will help you enjoyably fulfill current fitness recommendations *and* the weekly goals outlined in the 7-Day Vitality Plan (see Chapter 12). These moves will not only add some spice to your new or typical routine, but can also help you look and feel more vibrant and energized, while keeping your heart, bones and muscles strong and your stress at bay. Choose the activities that are realistic and convenient for you to do. The key is to make a commitment to move more—and sit less—from the start, and to create a home and work environment and a schedule that support your efforts.

VITAL MOVES

I walk my younger son to school and then walk home (twenty-six blocks in total) almost daily, and I power walk (especially in the park, often with a friend), hula hoop, jump rope and weight train. Occasionally, I dance (tap and Zumba), ice-skate (one of my true loves), play basketball, tennis or golf, or hike (which I *love*) with my husband and sons. To find the right moves for you, think about what you enjoy when it comes to fitness. Do you like crowded or small fitness classes? Do you prefer to go to a gym and use machines or to work out in the great outdoors or in the comfort of your own home? Do you like exercising to music, or do you prefer calm and quiet? Do you like to work out with friends or on your own? Find activities that you enjoy and that you look forward to. It's fun to experiment with a variety of fitness classes with different instructors as a way to find those that you enjoy and that fit into your schedule. Making the effort is well worth it.

If you're wondering which moves are better for vitality, here's my thought. While it's true that some activities enable you to burn more calories than others or work your heart and muscles harder (for example, climbing stairs is much tougher than walking), what matters most is that you find activities *you* like to do and just do them! Starting slowly and easing your way into your new, active lifestyle is also critical to reduce injury risk and avoid burnout. Be sure to vary your routine at least every few weeks to stimulate different muscles and reduce the boredom factor. And never start any fitness program without clearance from your doctor, just to play it safe!

Wondering when the best time to exercise is? Whenever you can do it is the best time to do it. But if your schedule is flexible, exercising early in the day is a great way to stock up on physical and mental energy. Although late-day exercise is better than no exercise, working up a sweat too close to bedtime raises your body temperature and may make it tougher to fall asleep, whereas allowing a few hours between exercise and sleep for your body to cool can help you fall asleep faster.

Although the 7-Day Vitality Plan outlined in Chapter 12 provides a weekly template that includes fitness, laughter, reflection and, of course, sleep—all key components to help you work toward the 7 Pillars of Vitality—it's up to you to create your own fitness path, because only you know what you *want* to do, what you realistically *can* do, and what you're *willing* to do to achieve and maintain fitness and reap its many benefits.

In the following pages, you'll find some Vital Moves to help you get started.

WALK THIS WAY

Walking is one of the best vitality boosters, and it's so easy—you just put one foot in front of the other! You can power walk as part of your exercise regime (I've proudly walked two half marathons, and training for them kept me very motivated to make it to the park often), or simply make it a point to walk rather than take a car, bus, taxi or train to get from place to place. Wearing a pedometer or other tracking device can keep you on course and motivate you to set and achieve daily and weekly goals.

ENJOY RECESS

Remember how you used to love the sound of the school bell ringing for recess? Rediscover the joys of play and having fun while moving. Play has been shown to improve mood and increase vitality. You can play tag or ball with your children (or nieces and nephews or friends' kids), hula hoop (hoopnotica.com has some great hoops to choose from), jump rope (a great quick and easy aerobic workout), skip or play hopscotch.

GO GREEN

Take your workout outdoors! Whether you walk, bike, run, do push-ups or crunches, or do yoga or Pilates or any combination of moves, there's evidence that taking your routine outside can give you a psychological boost, making your workout that much better. (Just be sure to check the weather and dress appropriately, and wear plenty of sunscreen to protect your face and other parts from the sun, cold and wind.) In a review published in *Environmental Science and Technology* in 2011, researchers noted that adults reported feeling more revitalized, energetic and engaged and less tense, confused, angry and depressed while exercising outdoors compared with exercising indoors. Subjects also reported that they enjoyed outdoor activity and felt more satisfied with it than with indoor activity. They also were more likely to repeat the activity in the future. In another study, this one published in 2011 in the *American Journal of Health Behavior,* researchers determined that while biking or walking alone indoors made subjects feel more relaxed and calm, compared with doing those activities while listening to music or with a friend, exercising outdoors was more enjoyable overall and made subjects feel less tense and stressed.

STRIKE A POSE

Yoga and tai chi have been linked with countless mental and physical benefits. A review published in the *Journal of Alternative and Complementary Medicine* in 2010 analyzed twelve studies in which yoga was compared to other forms of exercise (such as walking, running, dancing or stationary biking) and found that in both healthy and unhealthy subjects, yoga was as effective, if not more effective, at improving blood glucose and lipid levels, easing fatigue and pain, and providing other health benefits. And an eight-week tai chi intervention improved antioxidant capacity and reduced cardiovascular risks in premenopausal and postmenopausal sedentary women, according to a study that appeared in the *Journal of Aging Research* in 2011.

GO FOR A BURST

Short on time? Then why not walk, run, bike (on a stationary bike) or jump rope as fast as you possibly can for a minute or so? Doing interval training—alternating intense exertion with lighter exertion—a few times a week can increase your calorie burn, boost your mood, strengthen your heart and provide other benefits, especially when you squeeze it in between all your other activities.

If you don't have thirty- or sixty-minute blocks of time for exercise, just "take ten." Divide your workout into three or six ten-minute bursts. According to the American Heart Association, breaking up activity in this way offers similar health and weight-loss benefits to doing thirty continuous minutes.

7 Moves You Can't Refuse

If you're looking to reduce stress, develop core strength and tone your belly—and your whole body—here's a quick and easy twenty-minute body-strengthening sequence, created by celebrity yoga and Pilates instructor Kristin McGee. According to McGee, "The sequence is basic enough for anyone to do, and solid enough for even the most advanced person to get a good workout, because every move works the entire body." You can use one or more of these moves as part of the "Lift It" component of the 7-Day Vitality Plan, as outlined in Chapter 12.

1. **Cat/Cow:** Strengthens the deep abdominal muscles and lower back. Also stretches the entire back, neck and shoulders. Begin on all fours, with your hands under your shoulders and your knees under your hips. Inhale, lifting your head and hips while arching your back as you pull your shoulder blades together. Keep your lower abs engaged to protect your lower back. Exhale. Round your body up toward the ceiling, scooping your belly while feeling a lift from your internal abdominal muscles. Tuck your head and tailbone, as if trying to bring them together underneath you like a scared cat. Continue rounding and arching for five to eight breaths.

2. **Knee to Nose:** Tones lower and deep abdominal muscles, back and hips. With your back rounded, inhale as you use your lower abs to pull your right knee toward your nose, and then exhale and extend the leg straight back as your head comes back to neutral. Do this five to eight times with each side.

3. **Bird Dog:** Tones all abdominal muscles, waist, back and hips. From all fours, reach your right arm forward at ear level and extend your left leg straight back at hip height. Imagine you are balancing a cup of water on your lower back and another on your upper back, between your shoulder blades. Brace your core and hold for thirty to sixty seconds (remember to breathe!). Without spilling your imaginary water, return your arm and leg to the floor. Repeat on the opposite side. That's one rep. Do three to five reps.

continued on page 168

4. **Forearm Plank:** Tones center, deep and side abdominal muscles, back, waist, hips, legs, butt, arms and shoulders. Lie on your belly with your legs straight, your elbows under your shoulders and bent to ninety degrees, your forearms on the floor. Tighten your abs, press your hands into the floor and tuck your toes. Lift your hips so your body hovers ten to twelve inches above the floor. Your body should form a straight line from your head to your heels. Tighten an imaginary seat belt around your waist as you continue to draw your low belly in. Hold for forty-five to sixty seconds.

5. **Downward-Facing Dog:** Works the entire body, stretches hamstrings, hips, lower back and shoulders, and strengthens arms, abdominal muscles, legs and core. From all fours, tuck your toes under and lift your hips up and back, straightening out your legs to form an upside-down V. Press firmly into your hands and bring your torso back toward your upper thighs. If your hamstrings are tight, bend your knees slightly. Hold for five to eight breaths. Come down to rest in a child's pose* and then have a seat.

6. **Boat:** Tones deep abs, side abs, waist, inner thighs and pelvic floor. Sit tall with your knees bent and your feet flat on the floor. Without rounding your lower back, lean back slightly and lift your legs in the air, keeping your knees bent. Keep your shins parallel to the floor, or make it tougher by extending your legs straight out at an angle. Reach your arms forward with your palms turned inward. Pull your belly button to your spine and lift out of your lower back, pressing your shoulders down and away from your ears as you hold for thirty to sixty seconds. Repeat two more times.

7. **Bridge:** Tones buttocks, hips, core, stretches shoulders and opens up the chest for deeper breathing and relaxation. Lying on your back, place your feet flat on the mat hip-width apart. Press into your feet and lift up your hips. Clasp your hands under your back, and move your chest toward your chin. Try to tuck your tailbone under slightly, engage your hamstrings and buttocks, and press your feet firmly to the floor. Hold here for three to five breaths, and then lower down and repeat two more times.

*Rest your hips back on your heels (toes flat) and let your forehead drop to the floor. You can extend your arms forward out in front of you, palms resting on the mat, or rest your hands back alongside your waist.

For more information, visit Kristin McGee's website: www.kristinmcgee.com/meet-kristin.

FUELING FOR FITNESS

To help you eat before, during or after your exercise routine, here are some tips from my good friend and colleague Tara Gidus, MS, RD, sports nutritionist and team dietitian for the Orlando Magic:

FUELING BEFORE

- Stay hydrated all day long. Have a big glass or two of water when you wake up in the morning and drink plenty of fluids throughout the day to stay hydrated. Drink two cups of water two hours before exercise, too.

- Eat a meal or snack within two hours of exercise to prevent low blood sugar during your workout. Pre-workout meals should be lower in fat, low fiber, and bland to prevent gastrointestinal problems.

- Before your workout, avoid greasy and fried foods, anything spicy or unusual for you, and foods that have been known to upset your stomach.

FUELING DURING

The role of nutrition during a workout is twofold: it prevents low blood sugar and helps maintain hydration. Since even a 2 percent loss in body fluid can hamper your performance, it's important to drink fluids during exercise to optimize your workout. Drink four to eight ounces of fluids every fifteen to twenty minutes during your workout. Sports drinks and/or simple carbohydrates that are easy to digest, such as bananas, dried figs, energy bars and gels, are recommended when your workout lasts longer than one hour. This will help prevent low blood sugar and keep your working muscles energized.

FUELING AFTER

- Eat foods that are high in carbohydrates within thirty minutes of ending your workout to refuel depleted muscle glycogen. This improves recovery and future performance and can decrease muscle soreness. If you're not too hungry afterward, have a cup of low-fat chocolate milk, a great recovery beverage because of its 4:1 ratio of carbohydrates to protein and its sodium content. Eat a meal with carbohydrates and protein within two hours of your workout to replenish energy stores and maintain lean muscle mass.

■ Eat foods that are rich in antioxidants, such as fruits and vegetables or smoothies made with them, and omega-3 fatty acids (found in fatty fish, such as salmon and halibut, and in "little" fish, such as sardines and anchovies) to reduce inflammation and decrease muscle soreness, thereby improving recovery.

Staying active by walking more and finding activities you enjoy doing solo or with others who have similar interests, and sitting less are just some of the strategies that can help you achieve and maintain the 7 Pillars of Vitality. Getting fit, and reaping the many benefits being fit provides, is not about starting or stopping being active; it's about finding ways to incorporate more activity into your daily life. Using the Vital Moves and Stressipes in this chapter, and visiting a few of my favorite fitness websites listed below, can provide you with motivation and resources to help you get and stay active and fit for life.

American College of Sports Medicine: www.acsm.org

American Council on Exercise: www.acefitness.org

The President's Challenge: www.presidentschallenge.org

VITAL RELAXATION

Welcome to Sleepless in Stressville. If your life feels like it is stuck in overdrive, then you've probably endured your share of sleepless nights. I know I have. Recently, my ten-year-old son had some sleep troubles—almost every night—for about a month. At first, he'd gently nudge me, and I'd let him sleep with us. Unfortunately, he's a restless sleeper to begin with, and at one point he was literally on top of me—and he weighs almost seventy pounds! After a few rough nights, I decided to "sleepwalk" him back to his bed, praying we both wouldn't tumble down the dark staircase. After more than a week of this routine, he no longer woke me, but he would come into our room and settle down to sleep on the sofa there. These nightly visits and the lack of sleep really took a toll on me. It made me worry, even more than usual, about how I was going to get through my lengthy to-do lists. Despite exercising nearly every day to get some energy, I felt extremely frazzled, and all I thought about was getting some caffeine. I started craving foods that I knew would only drain my vitality.

Sound familiar? I bet it does, especially if you have young or school-age children, or a teen who comes home at all hours of the night, well after you've tried to settle into bed. Or maybe you have so much on your mind (work, money, relationships) that it's difficult to fall asleep, and it's even harder to wake the next morning. Talk about brain drain!

It's no surprise that an estimated 35 percent of women, especially as they get older, report difficulty falling asleep, night waking and oversleeping—which are some of the most prevalent symptoms they experience when stressed, according to the American Psychological Association's 2012 *Stress in America* survey. Disrupted sleep also topped the list of symptoms among the women who took my Vitality Survey, with 65 percent of them saying they have trouble sleeping. Unfortunately, not getting enough quality sleep leaves you more vulnerable to, and less able to cope with, chronic stress, let alone the stress experienced every day, and it sets up a vicious cycle that makes you feel like you're dangling off a ledge.

HOW LACK OF SLEEP DILUTES YOUR VITALITY

A too-busy lifestyle disrupts sleep in many ways, making it difficult to fall asleep, causing you to wake up in the middle of the night with stressful thoughts racing through your head, or leaving you tossing and turning all night. And a lack of sleep for whatever reason—being a new (or worried) parent, having a looming deadline, experiencing relationship woes, or having perimenopausal or menopausal night sweats—does a number on your vitality. You may as well be pressing the Fast-Forward button on the aging process. A lack of sleep makes you look and feel ragged, puts you in a foul mood, brings on a serious case of brain fog and shifts your immune function into low gear, and as if that weren't enough, it can be an absolute disaster for your waistline.

SKIN WOES

A lack of sleep prevents your body from performing many of the restorative, rejuvenating processes that typically take place while you snooze. You wake up with dark circles under your eyes, which make you look more tired than you feel. When sleep deprivation becomes chronic, it pumps up the production of the stress hormone cortisol in your body. That makes you more prone to breakouts, shifts skin repair into slow motion, and leaves your skin looking duller, less vibrant and more wrinkled. And don't think that you can fix these problems with a quick trip to the cosmetics counter. A lack of sleep reduces the effectiveness of all those pricey products.

ZAPPED ENERGY

Routinely skimping on sleep leaves you feeling exhausted in every way. Physically, you drag yourself around, and you are far more likely to hit the couch than hit the gym. Mentally, it isn't much better. Research shows that if you don't get adequate sleep, you're more likely to have trouble paying attention, concentrating, problem solving, reasoning and staying alert. You're also more prone to memory problems. If you've ever walked into a room after a sleepless night and then wondered, "Why did I come in here?" you know what I'm talking about. A lack of sleep also lowers your libido, which means you won't be getting the benefit of all those stress-relieving, feel-good chemicals that are released during orgasm.

MOODY BLUES

A single restless night can make you feel sad, angry or irritated. But when sleep eludes you night after night, your moods just get worse. In fact, chronic insomnia is associated with depression. Talk about sad bed partners. A study published in *Sleep* in 2007 tracked more than twenty-five thousand Norwegian adults for eleven years and found that those who had chronic insomnia were more likely to have anxiety and depression than those who didn't have trouble sleeping.

WEIGHT GAIN

Studies suggest that too little sleep wreaks havoc with two hormones that regulate your appetite—leptin and ghrelin—meaning that, when you don't sleep well, you feel hungrier, eat more and choose more nutrient-poor foods. A 2006 study in the *American Journal of Epidemiology* determined that women who slept five hours or less per night gained the most weight and were more likely to become obese than women who slept six or more hours. One of my blog readers, Lauren, who responded to my Vitality Survey, doesn't need scientific studies to confirm that skimping on sleep translates into more stress and weight gain. "I really notice that when I'm stressed and can't sleep, I wake up starving, and I eat things that I normally wouldn't, like the kids' Pop-Tarts, doughnuts, or leftover pizza for breakfast," she wrote. "If I don't sleep well for several days in a row, my stress gets out of control, and I start to gain weight fast."

When a Craving Strikes, Wait it Out.

According to New York City-based psychologist Lisa Morse, PhD, cravings are time limited: they tend to increase over a relatively short period of time, peak and eventually start to diminish. When a craving hits, Morse recommends waiting twenty minutes to see if the urge passes, allowing you to make a better choice. She says, "Ask yourself if you really want that cigarette, cookie, or drink." As you wait for the craving to go away, Morse recommends practicing stress-reduction techniques, such as breathing, meditation and progressive muscle relaxation; reaching out to someone to share feelings; listening to music, reading a book or watching a show you like; changing your environment (going for a walk); or taking a hot bath, lighting candles or having a cup of herbal tea to soothe and relax yourself.

On the flip side, some women, like my blog follower Renée, tend to oversleep when they're stressed. She sent this comment to me: "When things get crazy in my life, I just want to eat comfort foods and hibernate." And that's no good for your figure, either. In a 2008 study published in *Sleep,* researchers reported that adults who slept for nine or ten hours every night were 21 percent more likely to become obese over a six-year period than those who slept between seven and eight hours. Clearly, getting too little *or* too much sleep can take its toll.

INCREASED STRESS

Sleep deprivation causes your body to churn out greater quantities of the stress hormone cortisol, which only piles on stress. In a 2005 study in the *Journal of Endocrinology and Metabolism,* researchers from Northwestern University reported that sleep deprivation activates the hypothalamic-pituitary-adrenal (HPA) axis, one of the main neuroendocrine stress systems, and it causes the body to react more strongly to stress.

Redress Your Stress

No matter what stresses you—money, work, the economy, relationships, family responsibilities, your health or that of family members, or several things at once—learning how to perceive stressors differently and cope in a more healthful, proactive and positive way will add years to your life and life to your years. Here are five research-based healthy techniques to help you reduce short- and long-term stress, courtesy of the American Psychological Association's "Five Tips to Help Manage Stress":

1. **Take a break from the stressor.** It may seem difficult to get away from a big work project, a crying child or a growing credit card bill. But when you give yourself permission to step away from it, you allow yourself time to do something else, which can help you gain a new perspective or practice techniques to feel less overwhelmed. It's important to not avoid your stress (those bills have to be paid sometime), but even just taking twenty minutes to care for yourself can be helpful.

2. **Exercise.** The research keeps growing—exercise benefits your mind just as well as your body. We keep hearing about the long-term benefits of a regular exercise routine. But even a twenty-minute walk, run, swim or dance session in the midst of a stressful time can give an immediate effect that can last for several hours.

3. **Smile and laugh.** Our brains are interconnected with our emotions and facial expressions. When people are stressed, they often hold a lot of the stress on their face. So laughs or smiles can help relieve some of that tension and improve the situation.

4. **Get social support.** Call or email a friend. Sharing your concerns or feelings with another person helps to relieve stress. But it's important that the person to whom you talk is someone you trust and someone who can understand and validate you. If family is a stressor, for example, it may not alleviate your stress if you share your woes with one of your family members.

5. **Meditate.** Meditation and mindful prayer help the mind and body to relax and focus. Mindfulness can help you see new perspectives and develop self-compassion and forgiveness. When practicing a form of mindfulness, you can release emotions that may have been causing the body physical stress. Research has shown that much like exercising, even meditating briefly can confer immediate benefits.

REDUCED HEALTH AND WELL-BEING

Lack of sleep depresses your immune system and leaves you prone to colds and flu bugs, but even worse, it puts you at a higher risk for serious diseases and conditions, including an early death. In 2011, researchers reported in the *European Heart Journal* that adults who sleep less than six hours a night have a 48 percent greater chance of having a heart attack or dying from a heart attack, and a 15 percent greater chance of having a stroke or dying from a stroke.

FOOD FIXES AND STRESSIPES FOR MORE RESTFUL SLEEP

Are you tired of stress-induced sleep problems? Head to your kitchen for relief! No, I don't mean you should raid the fridge at midnight. What I mean is that knowing which foods and beverages to choose, how much to consume and when to eat and drink them may very well mean the difference between tossing and turning or sleeping soundly. Perhaps even more important, knowing which foods and drinks to limit or avoid can be your ticket to a good night's sleep. That's because many foods and beverages act as natural sedatives, while others are potent energizers.

AMINO ACIDS

If your stress is keeping you up at night, then you might want to get a little more cozy with tyrosine and tryptophan, two key amino acids found in many protein-rich foods (see Chapter 5). I know, it's kind of a mouthful, but these nutrients are found in many delicious foods that are probably already in your kitchen. And when you see how they can promote sleep, you'll probably join their fan club, too.

TYROSINE

Tyrosine is an amino acid that acts as a natural energizer and is found in many high-protein foods, including chicken, turkey, fish, soybeans, avocados, nuts and seeds, and dairy products. Consuming a protein-rich meal can raise tyrosine levels in the blood and the brain and cause neurons to make norepinephrine, a stress hormone and neurotransmitter, and dopamine, a neurotransmitter. Together, they promote alertness and activity, which is *not* what you want right before you hit the sack.

Pump Up the Tyres—Early!

To promote better sleep, consume most of your tyrosine-rich protein during the day, and taper it off after midday and as you get closer to bedtime. For example, top low-fat cottage cheese with a banana and pumpkin seeds for breakfast. At lunch, have a colorful salad with turkey breast, avocado and a little cheese. At dinner, have some pasta loaded with veggies and one or two small chicken meatballs.

In general, all protein-rich foods help keep you full and help maintain steady blood sugar levels throughout the day. And when you're sleep deprived, they're especially important to keep you energized so you can power through your day.

Are you tired all the time? Consider having your doctor check your thyroid levels. Tyrosine is needed by the body to make active thyroid hormones. Low blood levels of tyrosine have been associated with an underactive thyroid, which can cause fatigue.

TRYPTOPHAN

You've probably heard that eating tryptophan-rich turkey is what makes you feel like you need a nap after your big Thanksgiving feast. But what is tryptophan, and how does it affect sleep? Tryptophan is a naturally occurring amino acid found in protein-rich foods, including chicken, turkey, fish, eggs, milk, soybeans and tofu, and nuts and seeds. As you learned in Chapter 5, tryptophan helps make the "feel-good," sleep-inducing neurotransmitter serotonin. Tryptophan also is involved in the production of melatonin, a sleep-promoting hormone made in the brain.

Although eating tryptophan-rich foods won't raise brain serotonin levels (remember, tryptophan needs carbohydrates to gain entry into the brain to produce serotonin), eating small amounts throughout the day gives the body the foundation for creating more serotonin and maintaining adequate serotonin stores when you fall asleep. This all adds up to a better chance of staying asleep!

Take a Day Tryp.

Eat small amounts of tryptophan-rich protein throughout the day to improve your chances of falling asleep and staying asleep at night. For instance, try a hard-boiled egg as part of your breakfast, have some salmon with your lunch, and sprinkle some sunflower seeds on a bowl of butternut squash soup as part of your dinner.

CALM YOURSELF DOWN WITH CARBS

As discussed in Chapter 3, carbs have been unfairly blamed for causing everything from belly fat to diabetes. But starchy carbs, especially the whole-grain, high-fiber kind, aren't the enemy. In fact, eating moderate amounts of carbohydrate-rich foods—think whole-wheat pasta, a baked potato, oatmeal or low-sugar, ready-to-eat cereal—within a few hours of bedtime can help with the absorption of tryptophan in the brain to produce sleep-inducing serotonin. Elizabeth Somer, MA, RD, author of *Eat Your Way to Happiness,* says, "To maximize the serotonin boost, have a snack that contains 30 grams (about an ounce) of carbohydrate, such as 4 cups of air-popped popcorn, a 100 percent whole-wheat English muffin with two teaspoons of jam, or 9 Triscuits 30 minutes before you need to relax or go to bed."

Out of Sight, Out of Your Mouth!

Keep foods that you can't say no to and/or tend to overeat out of your home (and out of your desk drawer at work). If you're tempted by some of the foods your family members enjoy, like chips, cookies or candy, store them on a high shelf behind closed doors to minimize temptation.

A study published in the *American Journal of Clinical Nutrition* in 2007 found that eating a carbohydrate-based, high-glycemic index (GI) meal four hours before bedtime helped people fall asleep faster than eating a low-GI meal with a low-protein content.

Cozy Up with Carbs in the Evening.

When you are stressed and have trouble sleeping, focus on carbs for dinner. Whole-wheat pasta with veggies or a brown rice stir-fry are nutritious options. And enjoy a small handful—just one!—of jelly beans or a favorite carbohydrate-rich sweet treat before bedtime.

Let me be clear here. I'm not saying that it's okay to gobble down a big bag of pretzels or half a loaf of bread by itself in one sitting. According to sleep expert Michael Grandner, PhD, "High-carb meals don't need to be excessive to be effective." Too much carbohydrate at a meal, for example, can lead to an unhealthy spike in insulin levels. Grandner says, "A small pasta dish with some Italian bread is one thing, but people might get the idea that *more* carbs is better—and that's not the case. Think *high-quality* carbs in moderation." (Warning! If you have diabetes, it is generally not recommended to eat high-glycemic meals.)

To Reduce Mindless Eating, Follow the Food Rule.

To reduce nighttime or anytime noshing when you're not hungry, make it a rule to eat only in the kitchen, at the table or on a countertop, except during special occasions, such as when you have friends over for cocktails or to watch a ball game.

HOW WHAT YOU DRINK AFFECTS YOUR SLEEP

What you drink, and when you drink, can have an impact on your ability to fall asleep and have a sound, restorative sleep.

ALCOHOL

Having even one nightcap has been shown to disrupt the restorative power of sleep. And it isn't just what you drink right before you hit the sack. Those few drinks with coworkers or friends at "not so happy hour"—and let's not forget all that extra food you may eat while you drink—also can keep you from getting a restful sleep.

Women who drink not only may suffer when it comes to sleep, but also can be at increased risk for alcohol disorders, including binge drinking (see Chapter 2 for more on drinking)—especially when under duress. It's also important to understand that alcohol affects you much more as you age than it did when you were younger. So, after having just a drink or two, you may be far more impaired than you think.

But for many women, the mere thought of giving up wine or cocktails ratchets up their levels of stress and anxiety. At lunch one day I was telling my friend Marni about all the research I'd uncovered about alcohol, sleep issues and the many other ways alcohol saps us of our vitality (see Vitality Check: Does More Drinking Equal Less Sleeping? on page 181). Marni looked at me and said, "Please don't take away Mr. Pinot! He's my best friend!"

But when I asked her how well she was sleeping, she confessed that she's a "terrible" sleeper who typically falls asleep easily but then wakes up in the middle of the night. So I convinced Marni to try giving up wine for one week. When I called to check in on Marni on her first night without Mr. Pinot, she said, "I don't like you very much right now, Elisa!" Ouch! That hurt. But I encouraged her to stick with it. By the end of the week, she told me that she had slept through the night the past three nights, and she hadn't done that in years!

Eventually, Marni decided to let Mr. Pinot back into her life, but only on an occasional basis, and she quickly noticed that on the nights she drank, she would wake up at 2:00 or 3:00 a.m. She says she isn't ready to kick Mr. Pinot to the curb completely, but at least now she knows how wine affects her sleep, appearance, moods and stress levels. She now feels empowered about when to drink and when to avoid it. And with the Stressipes in this chapter (and in Chapter 9), she is able to sleep better and minimize the damage the day after a wine-tasting event or a night out with her girlfriends.

Does More Drinking Equal Less Sleeping?

If you "need" a drink or two to unwind, you may want to rethink that strategy. While drinking may help you zonk out initially, research shows that alcohol will eventually disrupt sleep and increase wakefulness—especially in women. A 2011 study published in *Alcoholism: Clinical and Experimental Research* found that women who drank alcohol one to two and a half hours before bedtime got less sleep, spent more time in bed *not* sleeping and woke up more times than women who didn't drink. And when alcohol keeps you up during the second half of the sleep cycle, it can lead to daytime fatigue. (See Chapter 9 for Stressipes to help you cut back on alcohol.)

CAFFEINE AND CAPPUCCINOS

When we don't get enough sleep, so many of us reach for a cup of coffee, tea, soda or a caffeinated energy drink (see Chapter 9 for more information about drinks). For most women, having one or two cups of a caffeinated beverage in the morning won't interfere with sleep. It's when you're so stressed that you're drinking coffee or Diet Coke all day long and into the evening (okay, I've been guilty of this one!) that it can keep you from falling asleep or cause you to wake up in the middle of the night. The next morning you feel like a zombie, so you reach for your caffeine fix to jump-start your day, and the vicious cycle starts all over again.

You don't need piles of scientific studies to know that caffeine can have profound effects on sleep and wake function. Did you know that caffeine is considered a *psychoactive* substance? That means it literally is a *drug* that crosses the blood-brain barrier and affects brain function, as well as mood, cognition and behavior. That's a lot of bang for that two-dollar cup of joe! Caffeine blocks sleep-inducing chemicals in the brain, fooling our brains into thinking we don't need sleep. When we're sleep deprived, that delicious latte or refreshing Diet Coke pumps up the production of adrenaline, manipulates our mental state and restores cognitive performance. Unfortunately, lab studies have also documented how caffeine may disrupt subsequent sleep and result in daytime sleepiness.

To prevent caffeine-induced sleeping troubles, avoid caffeinated beverages in the afternoon and evening. And don't forget to limit other sources of caffeine, including over-the-counter medications (such as Excedrin) and—dare I say it—large amounts of caffeine-containing chocolate and foods made with chocolate.

Stressipe

When It Comes to Caffeine, Be an Early Bird.

If you're having trouble sleeping but need your caffeine fix (it can be a good pick-me-up for the sleep deprived), stick to one or two eight-ounce cups of coffee or tea, one can of soda or one bottled iced tea (preferably without added sugar) before 2:00 p.m. or so. If you still have trouble sleeping, taper your caffeine consumption slowly to minimize withdrawal effects, especially rebound headaches.

How do you kick the caffeine habit? Go cold turkey or taper off? If you're going cold turkey, you may experience headaches, fatigue, sleepiness, an inability to focus or concentrate, irritability, depression, anxiety or even flu-like symptoms. Michal Kuhar, chief of the division of neuroscience at Yerkes National Primate Research Center, says, "Withdrawal symptoms can start from twelve to twenty hours after your last cup of coffee and peak about two days later and can last about as long as a week."

If you want to give up caffeinated beverages, taper your intake gradually by drinking smaller servings at the same time each day to minimize withdrawal symptoms. For example, if you drink two twenty-ounce bottles of caffeinated soda per day, taper to two twelve-ounce cans, then only one can at lunch over the course of a few weeks. If you're a coffee lover, you may want to substitute a portion of decaf coffee for regular in each cup and gradually shift to decaf only. But remember that decaf coffees and teas still contain some caffeine. (See page 148 for Stressipes to help you curb caffeine intake.)

Good-Bye, Diet Coke! Breaking Up Is Hard To Do

I am well acquainted with the perils of caffeine withdrawal. As I was writing this book, I realized that my thirty-plus-year habit of drinking Diet Cokes (several cans a day for the last ten years or so) probably wasn't helping my energy levels or stress levels and might have contributed to occasional sleeping problems (and might lead to health issues, like metabolic syndrome or kidney problems, down the road). One Saturday morning, when I realized I had no Diet Coke in my refrigerator, I decided then and there to quit my habit once and for all. I didn't buy my beloved Diet Coke on my way home from my morning power walk, and I didn't drink one while watching my older son's basketball practice or when my family grabbed dinner out. Yes, I thought about it all day long. I also felt a little moody, and by the afternoon, I had developed a dull, throbbing headache. But I knew that moderation would not work for me, so I went cold turkey and just suffered. I blogged about my effort to quit Diet Coke and told friends and relatives to stay accountable, which really helped me stay on course.

After twelve days, I stopped suffering from headaches and the midday fatigue, and my moodiness went away. I still missed my old friend on an emotional level. After all, thirty years is a long-term relationship—a lot longer than I've been with my husband! And Diet Coke had helped me through so much over the years: cramming for finals in college, coping with deaths of loved ones, planning my wedding, getting through crazy days with my sons, and yes, meeting book deadlines. With each passing day, though, I got a little more used to seeing a bottle of water on my desk instead of that old familiar silver and red can. And now, more than two years later, I haven't had any Diet Coke (except for a few sips, which I didn't like). Breaking up with a bad habit isn't easy, but if I can say good-bye to Diet Coke, then maybe you can overcome your less-than-healthy habits, too.

CHERRIES AND CHERRY JUICE

Should you eat tart cherries or swig tart cherry juice for a sweet slumber? Touted for their anti-inflammatory and antioxidant properties, cherries and cherry juice have garnered headlines as go-to sleep aids. But where's the proof? A small study published in the *European Journal of Nutrition* in 2012 concluded that drinking tart cherry juice led to significant increases in melatonin levels, sleep duration and sleep quality in twenty healthy volunteers. Researchers found that when these subjects consumed two cups of tart cherry juice—one when they woke up and another before bed—for seven days, they slept thirty-nine minutes longer on average and spent significantly less awake time in bed compared to when they consumed a placebo beverage. The researchers believe these effects were due to the high melatonin content of the cherry juice.

The bottom line? While cherry juice may show some promise as a sleep aid, I'm skeptical. And I don't need to tell you that if you drink too much of anything too close to bedtime, you may very well need to wake up to use the bathroom in the night. But if it's great taste and health benefits you're after, tart cherries are a win-win. They are packed with tons of antioxidants, such as beta-carotene and vitamin C, and also boast potassium, magnesium, iron, fiber and folate. Emerging evidence suggests that besides their potential heart-health benefits, they may reduce inflammation, ease arthritis symptoms and reduce post-exercise pain. Nine cherries count as a half cup of fruit on the Vitality Diet. So enjoy them!

Do 'Em Or Ditch 'Em?

Can Melatonin-Rich Foods Mellow You Out?

Melatonin is a natural hormone that's part of the human sleep-wake cycle, also known as circadian rhythms. It's made by the body's pineal gland, a pea-size gland located just above the middle of the brain. The pineal gland is inactive during the day, but when the sun sets and the lights dim, the pineal gland party gets started and it begins to pump out melatonin, which makes us feel sleepy. Some health experts advocate eating foods containing melatonin as a way to promote relaxation, but the jury is still out on this theory. Even though melatonin-rich foods, such as tomatoes, olives, barley, rice and walnuts, can raise blood levels of melatonin after they're consumed, a 2012 review published in *Food and Nutrition Research* suggests that the vitamins and minerals in such foods may help the body naturally create melatonin. But some scientists say the melatonin in food doesn't get converted to melatonin in the brain and therefore won't help you get any shut eye. Still, many melatonin-rich foods are also rich in starchy carbs, which can affect serotonin levels and promote sleep, so feel free to do 'em and see if they help you settle down.

ALL THE RIGHT MOVES FOR BETTER SLEEP

Several studies (a few of which are discussed in Chapter 10) show that engaging in regular exercise—whether on a treadmill, on a hiking trail, in a dance class, on a tennis court or in the comfort of your own home—can help you sleep better.

Exercising regularly is one of the best things you can do to improve your sleep. To maximize your ability to fall asleep and to sleep deeply, exercise early in the day to give your body time to cool off and prime you for sleep. According to Dario Acuña-Castroviejo, MD, PhD, professor of physiology at the University of Granada in Spain, morning exercise is optimal for another reason, as well: "Normal melatonin levels start to rise between 9:00 p.m. and 10:00 p.m., and evening exercise can alter the melatonin production in the body (and thereby hinder sleep)."

REVITALIZE YOUR BEDROOM AND SLEEP ROUTINE

Did you know that your bedroom or your late-night habits could be preventing you from getting the restful sleep you need to pump up your vitality? Make sure your bedroom *oozes* sleep. Close the windows or listen to calming nature tunes if the sounds of traffic, loud neighbors or barking dogs keep you awake. Create a soothing bedtime routine to help you calm down and drift off to sleep. Take a warm bath to relax; several studies suggest it can help you have a deeper sleep.

STRESSIPES FOR A GOOD NIGHT'S REST

Here are some Stressipes to help you get your z's:

1. **Stressipe: Follow the Goldilocks rule in the bedroom.** A room that is either too hot or too cold can contribute to restlessness and lots of tossing and turning. But when the temperature is in the proper range (most experts suggest a room that's slightly cool), your core body temperature drops slightly, which induces sleepiness. Just be sure to wear layers and slip on your socks if you know the cooler temperature and your chilly feet distract you from sleeping when you settle into bed.

2. **Stressipe: Power down in the p.m.** Whether you're tethered to a DVR, laptop, tablet, game console or smartphone, power them down at least a half hour (ideally more) before you hit the sack. Place your gadgets far from your bedroom so you aren't tempted by the siren call of the beeps or the blinking lights that signal incoming—and, of course, *urgent*—messages. Although few studies have looked at the associations between late-night technology use and sleep, some suggest that it may be linked with excessive movement during sleep,

insomnia, depressed mood and altered brain function during the day. So instead of activating your mind at night, use bedtime to rest rather than text!

3. **Stressipe: Dim all the lights, sweet darling.** Do you sleep with a night-light, a glowing alarm clock or the TV on in the background? If your body is exposed to light at night, it produces less of the sleep-inducing hormone melatonin, and that can prevent you from getting that revitalizing sleep you need and deserve. So dim those bright lights (but be sure to keep a little light so you don't trip on a trip to the bathroom if nature calls overnight).

4. **Stressipe: Grab a nap.** Research shows that taking a midday power nap lasting ten to no more than thirty minutes can decrease stress, improve alertness and boost cognitive function. Set an alarm to prevent your power nap from turning into a snooze fest that disrupts your nighttime sleep cycle.

Take a Break to Meditate

Have you ever thought of meditating, or does the thought of taking time out of your oh-so-busy life make you sweat? My friend Rachel Begun, a registered dietitian and spokesperson for the Academy of Nutrition and Dietetics, had explored the idea of meditation to find work-life balance for years. She learned the basics but was inconsistent. She then made a commitment and meditates nearly every day. Rachel says, "Meditation has changed me. I sleep better, and my days are less stressful and calmer, smoother and easier. And, professionally, I am just as driven as before but find it easier to achieve my goals while enjoying life more. Best of all, I am a more loving, compassionate person."

WAKE UP—EVEN ON WEEKENDS

Another sad but true fact is that oversleeping can be detrimental to your emotional and physical well-being and has been associated with depression, obesity, headaches, back pain, heart disease, diabetes and even death. (Yes, you have a higher risk of dying if you sleep nine or more hours a night.) So set that alarm and try to sleep the same amount on weekdays and weekends. It's not easy, but it's a routine that is sure to help you get on and stay on a road to better, more restful sleep. Here are a few simple moves to help you put a stop to excess slumber:

- Place your alarm clock far enough away from you that you have to get out of bed to turn it off.

- Keep the shades open to allow natural light to enter your room in the morning.

- Taper your sleep gradually by shaving fifteen to thirty minutes off your normal sleep time each week.

Vital Rx

Relaxation

- Consume small amounts of protein foods throughout the day to lay the foundation for the creation of sleep-promoting serotonin.
- Have small servings of starchy carbs, especially when you want to relax and unwind or when bedtime draws near.
- Create and follow a consistent bedtime routine on weekdays and weekends to maximize your ability to fall asleep and stay asleep and to enhance the overall quality of your sleep.

PART THREE

VITALITY FOR LIFE

12

THE 7-DAY VITALITY PLAN

To help you get—and keep—the vitality boost you're looking for, I've designed a comprehensive, yet easy-to-follow 7-Day Vitality Plan based on the food, fitness and lifestyle principles and remedies outlined in Part II of this book. This jump-start plan includes a delicious menu, a Vital Foods List and a blueprint to help you incorporate fitness and other lifestyle strategies that will help you achieve and maintain the 7 Pillars of Vitality.

7 DAYS TO A NEW YOU

If you're looking for a quick fix for weight loss, you won't find that here. That's because achieving vitality is not about going on and off a restrictive, hard-to-follow diet. It's about finding sustainable balance in your food choices and overall lifestyle. The 7-Day Vitality Plan is designed to help you achieve slow and steady, rather than rapid, weight loss. Losing too much weight too fast can sap your vitality and sabotage your efforts by leaving you hungry and making you feel deprived, especially if you consume significantly fewer calories than you're used to and cut out too many of the foods you enjoy. So-called crash diets can exacerbate stress and heighten cortisol levels (two factors that actually contribute to weight gain and accelerated aging), and they can lead to the loss of lean muscle mass—the very thing you need to preserve to keep your metabolism revved up. And let's not forget that losing weight can also age your face and leave you with that unhealthy gaunt look—which is not a recipe for looking vibrant, is it? By incorporating all aspects of the 7-Day Vitality Plan, you'll be amazed at how, in just seven days, taking better care of yourself, which includes eating more nutrient-packed foods in appropriate portions throughout the day, not only can help you feel more energized and empowered, but can also help you better handle stress and get that coveted sleep you need, which will reduce crankiness and circles under your eyes and help you look and feel your very best.

YOUR VITALITY BLUEPRINT

To achieve the 7 Pillars of Vitality, it's important to not only nourish your body by eating nutritious foods in sensible portions, but also to take time each and every day to mindfully and purposefully care for your body and soul and to nurture your relationships with others. To provide you with some guidance, I've created a basic flexible blueprint you can use each and every day to help you incorporate Vital Foods, Vital Moves, Vital Relaxation and Vital Sleep into your lifestyle. Think of the blueprint as a framework for your life that provides just enough structure to help you stay energized and centered by day, and relaxed and settled by night. The beauty of the blueprint is that you can easily personalize the recommendations based on your own nutrient needs, interests and schedule.

Stressipe

Go Slow and Savor Your Food.

Chewing your food slowly and taking the time to savor and really taste your food, rather than shoveling it down, will help you enjoy each meal much more and will lessen the likelihood that you'll overeat. Pacing yourself can also give your brain a chance to register that it's satisfied.

VITAL FOODS

In the pages that follow, you'll find a Vital Foods List. In it you'll find a wide variety of nutritious, convenient options from the seven Vital Food categories, from which you can choose daily: Starchy Carbs, Fruits, Non-Starchy Vegetables, Proteins, Beans + Peas, Healthy Fats and Dairy. You'll also find a Treat Cheat Sheet if you cannot imagine life without some chocolate or wine or a handful of jelly beans—and why should you!

🍞 STARCHY CARBS

This category includes whole grains, starchy vegetables and refined grains. Choose four to five Starchy Carbs a day, emphasizing whole grains and non-starchy vegetable options.

Each item below = 1 Starchy Carb 🍞 (about 80–130 calories):

Whole Grains: Choose at least three a day.

- Brown or wild rice – ½ cup cooked or 1 ounce dry
- Bulgur – ½ cup cooked
- Corn tortilla – 1 (6" diameter)
- Oats or oatmeal – ½ cup cooked or 1 packet instant or 1 ounce (⅓ cup) dry
- Pita bread, whole-wheat – 1 small or ½ large
- Popcorn – 3 cups air-popped
- Pretzels, whole-wheat – 12 or 1 ounce
- Quinoa – ½ cup cooked
- Shredded Wheat, Spoon-Size – ½ cup
- Whole-grain cereal flakes – 1 cup
- Whole-grain granola, low-fat – ¼ cup
- Whole-grain pancakes, whole-wheat or buckwheat – 1 medium (4½" diameter) or 2 small (3" diameter)
- Whole-grain puffed cereal, wheat or rice – 2 cups
- Whole-grain tortilla chips – 7
- Whole-grain/whole-wheat bread – 1 slice

- Whole-grain/whole-wheat crackers – 5
- Whole-wheat bagel – ½ scooped or 1 "mini"
- Whole-wheat couscous – ½ cup cooked
- Whole-wheat English muffin – ½
- Whole-wheat flour tortillas – 1 small (6" diameter) or ½ large
- Whole-wheat hamburger bun – 1
- Whole-wheat pasta – ½ cup cooked or 1 ounce dry
- Whole-wheat roll – 1 small (2½" diameter)

Starchy Vegetables: Choose up to one or two a day.

- Corn, yellow or white – ½ cup kernels or ½ large ear (8–9" long)
- Cowpeas, field peas, or black-eyed peas, fresh (not dried) – ½ cup cooked
- Green lima beans – ½ cup
- Green peas – ½ cup
- Plantains – ½ cup
- Red potato – ½ cup baked or roasted, sliced, or 3 ounces
- Russet potato – ½ medium baked (2¼" or more diameter) or ½ cup cooked, sliced or mashed
- Sweet potato – ½ large baked (2¼" or more diameter) or ½ cup cooked, sliced or mashed
- Taro – ½ cup cooked
- Water chestnuts – ½ cup
- White potato – ½ medium (3 ounces), boiled or baked

Refined Grains: Choose no more than one or two a day (if desired).

- Bagel, plain or egg – ½ scooped or 1 "mini"
- Bread, white or French or sourdough or rye – 1 regular slice or 1 small slice French or 4 snack-size slices rye
- Corn bread – 1 small piece (2½" x 1¼" x 1¼")

- Cornflakes – 1 cup

- Couscous – ½ cup cooked

- Crackers – 7

- Croutons, nonfat, plain – ½ cup

- English muffin – ½

- Flour tortilla – 1 small (6" diameter)

- French bread, 1 large piece

- Granola, low-fat – ¼ cup*

- Pancakes, buttermilk or plain – 1 (4½" diameter) or 2 small (3" diameter)

- Panini bread, 1 slice

- Pasta – ½ cup cooked or 1 ounce dry

- Pita bread – 1 small or ½ large

- Potato chips, baked – 15 or 1 ounce

- Pretzels – 12 or 1 ounce

- Wheat germ – 3 Tbs

- White rice – ½ cup cooked or 1 ounce dry

*Check the ingredients list to see if it's whole grain.

🍎 FRUITS

This category includes fresh fruit, frozen fruit, dried fruit (made without added sugar) and 100 percent fruit juice. Choose one and a half Fruits a day.

Each item below = ½ Fruit 🍎 (about 50 calories):

- 100 percent fruit juice – ½ cup

- Apple – 1 extra small raw or ½ cup raw or cooked, sliced or chopped

- Applesauce, unsweetened – 1 snack container or 4 ounces

- Banana – ½ medium (7–8" banana)

- Blueberries – ½ cup

- Cantaloupe – 1 wedge (⅛ medium melon)

- Cherries, fresh – 5

- Cherries, pitted, fresh or frozen – about ⅓ cup

- Clementine – 1

- Dried fruit (apricots, plums, prunes, raisins, etc.) – ⅛ cup or 2 Tbs or ¾ ounce

- Grapefruit – ½ medium (4" diameter)

- Grapes, seedless – 16 or ½ cup whole or cut up

- Kiwi – 1 or ½ cup sliced

- Orange – 1 small (2⅜" diameter)

- Peach – 1 small (2" diameter)

- Pineapple – ½ cup chunks, sliced or crushed

- Plum – 1 large

- Raspberries, fresh or frozen – ½ cup

- Strawberries, fresh or frozen – 4 large or ½ cup whole, halved, or sliced

- Tangerine – 1 small

- Watermelon – 6 balls

NON-STARCHY VEGETABLES

This category includes fresh and frozen vegetables without added sugar or fat. Choose at least two Non-Starchy Vegetables a day.

Each item below = 1 Non-Starchy Vegetable 🥦 (about 40 calories):

- Asparagus – 4 medium spears, cooked

- Bean sprouts – 1 cup cooked

- Beets – 2 (2" diameter) or 1 cup

- Broccoli – 1 cup chopped florets or 3 spears 5" long, raw or cooked

- Brussels sprouts – ¾ cup, cooked

- Carrots – 1 cup raw or cooked, strips, slices, or chopped; or 2 medium/large or 1 cup baby (about 12)

- Cauliflower – 1 cup pieces or florets, raw or cooked

- Celery – 1 cup raw or cooked, diced or sliced; or 2 large stalks (11"–12" long)

- Cucumbers – 1 cup raw, sliced or chopped

- Green cabbage – 1 cup raw or cooked, chopped or shredded

- Green or wax beans – 1 cup cooked

- Green peppers – 1 large or 1 cup raw or cooked, chopped

- Greens (collards, mustard, turnip, kale) – 2 cups raw or 1 cup cooked

- Lettuce (iceberg or head) – 2 cups raw, shredded or chopped

- Mushrooms – 1 cup raw or cooked

- Onions – 1 cup raw or cooked, chopped

- Pumpkin – 1 cup cooked, mashed

- Raw leafy greens (romaine, watercress, dark green leafy lettuce, endive, escarole) – 2 cups raw

- Red pepper (and other sweet/bell peppers) – 1 large or 1 cup raw or cooked, chopped

- Spinach – 2 cups raw or 1 cup cooked

- Tomato sauce – ½ cup

- Tomatoes – 1 cup chopped or sliced, about 8 slices or 1 can red, ripe, no salt added

- Winter squash (acorn, butternut, hubbard, etc.) – ½ cup cooked, cubed

⬛ PROTEINS

This category includes lean beef and poultry (prepared without skin or breading), eggs, soybeans and soy foods, and nuts, nut butters, and seeds.* Choose about six Proteins a day.

Each item below = 1 Protein ⬛ (about 50 calories):

- Beef, lean – 1 ounce cooked

- Chicken or turkey, skinless – 1 ounce cooked

- Edamame – ¼ cup or 1 ounce

- Egg – 1 whole egg

- Egg whites – 3

- Fish or shellfish (salmon, tuna, sardines, cod, etc.) – 1 ounce cooked or canned

- Hummus – 2 Tbs

- Pork or ham, lean – 1 ounce cooked

- Soybeans – ¼ cup roasted

- Tempeh – 1 ounce cooked

- Tofu – ¼ cup (about 2 ounces) cooked

*Nuts, nut butters and seeds count as Proteins and Healthy Fats (see page 197, Healthy Fats).

Nuts, Nut Butters and Seeds: Choose two a day.

Each item below = 1 Protein 🌰 + 1 Healthy Fat 🫒 (about 100 calories):

- Almond butter – 1 Tbs

- Almonds – 12 whole or 2 Tbs chopped or ½ ounce

- Brazil nuts – 3 whole or ½ ounce

- Cashews – 13 whole

- Chestnuts – 3 whole or ½ ounce

- Chia seeds – 4–5 tsp or ½ ounce

- Flax seeds, ground – 2 Tbs or ½ ounce

- Hazelnuts – 10 whole or ½ ounce

- Macadamia nuts – 5–6 whole or ½ ounce

- Peanut butter – 1 Tbs

- Peanuts – 14 whole or 4–5 teaspoons chopped or ½ ounce

- Pecans – 5 whole or 10 halves

- Pine nuts – 4 tsp or ½ ounce

- Pistachios – 24 whole or ½ ounce

- Pumpkin seeds – 4–5 tsp or ½ ounce

- Sesame seeds – 2 Tbs or ½ ounce

- Sunflower seeds – 2 Tbs or ½ ounce

- Walnuts – 7 halves or 2 Tbs; or ⅛ cup chopped or ½ ounce

🫛 BEANS + PEAS

This category includes beans (excluding soybeans), peas and lentils. Choose at least six Beans + Peas (a total of 1½ cups) each week.

Each item below = 1 Beans + Peas 🫛 (about 50–75 calories):

- Baked/refried beans – ¼ cup

- Beans (black, kidney, pinto, white, etc.), canned – ¼ cup

- Chickpeas – ¼ cup cooked

- Cowpeas, field peas, black-eyed peas, mature, dried – ¼ cup cooked

- Lentils – ¼ cup cooked

- Lima beans, mature, dried – ¼ cup cooked

- Split pea, lentil or bean soup – ½ cup

- Split peas – ¼ cup cooked

🫘 HEALTHY FATS

This category includes oils, salad dressings and other added fats or fatty foods that contain mostly healthful monounsaturated and polyunsaturated fats and are used to enhance the flavor and add texture to other foods. (Nuts, nut butters and seeds, listed in the Protein group, also count as Healthy Fats.) Choose four to five Healthy Fats a day.

Each of the following = 1 Healthy Fat 🫘 (about 40 calories):

- Avocado – 2–3 thin slices (about 1 ounce or ⅕ medium)

- Guacamole – 4 tsp

- Margarine (trans fat–free) or vegetable oil spread – 1 tsp

- Mayonnaise – 1 tsp

- Mayonnaise-type salad dressing* – 1 Tbs

- Olives,* ripe, canned – 4 large

- Salad dressing (e.g., Italian or Thousand Island) – 2 Tbs

- Vegetable oils (olive, canola, corn, cottonseed, olive, peanut, safflower, soybean, sunflower, etc.) – 1 tsp

*Salad dressings and olives tend to be high in sodium, so keep portions small when you choose them.

DAIRY

This category includes low-fat and nonfat milk and yogurt, and cheese. Choose three Dairy items a day.

Milk and Yogurt:

Each of the following = 1 Dairy (80–140 calories):

- Buttermilk, low-fat or nonfat – 1 cup or 8 ounces

- Milk, flavored (chocolate, vanilla, strawberry), low-fat or nonfat – 1 cup or 8 ounces = 1 Dairy + a 50-calorie Treat*

- Milk, low-fat or nonfat – 1 cup or 8 ounces

- Regular or Greek yogurt, low-fat or nonfat plain – 1 cup or 1 regular container (8 ounces)

- Soy milk, calcium-fortified – 1 cup or 8 ounces

- Yogurt, flavored (with caloric sweeteners), low-fat or nonfat – 1 cup or 8 ounces= 1 Dairy + a 50- to 100-calorie Treat*

Cheese:

Each of the following = 1 Dairy (75–120 calories):

- American or other processed cheese – 1–1½ slices

- Blue cheese – ¼ cup crumbled or 1 ounce

- Cottage cheese, low-fat* – ½ cup

- Feta cheese – ¼ cup crumbled or 1 ounce

- Hard cheese (cheddar, mozzarella, Swiss, Parmesan, etc.) – one 1-ounce slice or ¼ cup shredded

- Parmesan cheese, grated – 4 level Tbs

- Ricotta cheese, part-skim – ½ cup

*Learn more about Treats on pages 199-201.

TREATS

Up to 150 calories in treats are included daily in the 7-Day Vitality Diet to satisfy your sweet tooth, your craving for salt or your desire for some bubbly. Below I've listed approximate 50- 100- and 150-calorie servings of various foods and beverages that contribute calories but few nutrients to your Vitality Diet. (Any mention of brand-name items should not be construed as an implied endorsement.) Use this list to make swaps in the 7-Day Vitality Meal Plan (see page 205). If you don't want to choose any Treats from this list, you can replace those extra calories with any food or drink you wish!

Stressipe

Have Your Treat While You Eat.

If there's a treat, such as chocolate or cookies, that you tend to overeat but would rather not give up (and why should you?), be sure to have it right after a meal or as part of a mid-morning or mid-afternoon snack instead of by itself. Having the meal or snack beforehand will likely fill you up and perhaps make you feel just as satisfied with a smaller portion than you might have otherwise.

Treat Cheat Sheet

Food	50 Calories	100 Calories	15-0 Calories
Sweets:			
Chips Ahoy! chocolate chip cookie	1	2	3
Dark chocolate Hershey Bar (1.25 ounces)	3-4 rectangles	6-8 rectangles	9-12 rectangles
Dark chocolate chips	1 Tbs	2 Tbs	3 Tbs
Fig Newtons	1	2	3
Frozen yogurt (Pinkberry)			½ level cup
Hershey's Kisses	2	4	6
Hoisin sauce*	4 tsp	8 tsp	12 tsp
Honey	1 Tbs	2 Tbs	3 Tbs
Honey mustard	1½ Tbs	3 Tbs	4½ Tbs

continued on page 202

Food	50 Calories	100 Calories	15-0 Calories
Jelly Belly jelly beans (small)	12	24	36
Jelly Belly jelly beans (large)	5	10	15
Ketchup	2½ Tbs	5 Tbs	7½ Tbs
M&M'S	15	30	45
Nutella	1½ tsp	1 Tbs	1½ Tbs
Oreo	1	2	3
Peanut M&M's	4	8	12
Snickers bar			½ regular-size bar
Sour Patch Kids	¼ bag	½ bag	¾ bag
Swedish Fish	2 regular/15 mini	4 regular/30 mini	6 regular/45 mini
Table sugar	1 Tbs	2 Tbs	3 Tbs
Tootsie Pops	1	2	3
Tootsie Rolls	2	4	6
Twix bar			1 (½ regular-size bar)
Twizzlers	1	2	3
Whipped cream	⅓ cup	⅔ cup	1 cup
Salty Snacks:			
Cheez-It crackers	4	8	12
Doritos	4	8	12
Fritos	10	20	30
Goldfish crackers	20	40	60
Popchips	10	20	30
Ritz crackers	3	6	9
Smartfood Popcorn	¼ cup	½ cup	¾ cup
Stacy's Pita Chips	4	8	12
Added Fats:			
Butter	1 tsp	2 tsp	1 Tbs
Coconut flakes	2 Tbs	4 Tbs	6 Tbs
Cream cheese	1 Tbs	2 Tbs	3 Tbs
Sour cream	2 Tbs	4 Tbs	6 Tbs
Drinks:			
Beer (light)	6 oz	12 oz	
Beer (regular)	4 oz	8 oz	12 oz

Food	50 Calories	100 Calories	15-0 Calories
Coca-Cola	4 oz	8 oz	12 oz
Distilled spirits		1½ oz	
Wine		5 oz	

*This is a high-sodium option.

Stressipe

To Curb a Craving, Just Chew It!

There's evidence that chewing gum can help squelch food cravings. In a study published in *Appetite* in 2011, researchers asked sixty subjects to rate their hunger, appetite and cravings for sweet and salty snacks for three hours after they ate lunch. The researchers found that when subjects chewed gum during the three hours, they ate 10 percent less of a snack than when they didn't chew gum. The researchers concluded that chewing gum for at least forty-five minutes promoted fullness and significantly suppressed hunger, appetite and cravings for snacks. If you want some treats as part of your Vitality Diet, go ahead and indulge, but if you want to prevent overeating, especially when you're not hungry, you may want to keep some sugarless gum in your arsenal.

VITAL MOVES

To maximize vitality, it's important to sit less and spend more time on your toes each and every day by simply walking more, engaging in moderate or vigorous activity at least five days a week and engaging in strength training at least twice a week.

Move It: Minimize the amount of time you spend sitting and aim to accumulate a total of ten thousand steps, or about five miles of walking, daily (see Appendix A to learn how to count the steps taken while doing your favorite activities). Wearing a pedometer or using an app that tracks your steps can help you stay on course. If you don't exercise regularly or consistently, build up to a minimum of thirty minutes of walking, biking, dancing or other moderate aerobic exercise on most days. You can do this in ten-minute bursts or all at once. Be sure to check with a physician before starting any exercise program. If you already exercise regularly and consistently, increase your time and/or intensity to stimulate your muscles even further and mix up your workout. Although it's important to take one or two "rest" days each week to repair muscles and reduce injury risk, make sure to sit less and move throughout each day to get the most vitality-boosting benefits. For more Vital Moves, see Chapter 10.

Lift It: Try to work all your key muscle groups with weights, fitness machines or resistance bands twice a week for twenty to forty minutes. Work with a certified personal trainer, use an exercise DVD or take a fitness class to learn the basics. You can find a reputable fitness trainer through the American College of Sports Medicine (ACSM), the American Council on Exercise (ACE) or the National Strength and Conditioning Association (NSCA).

VITAL RELAXATION

To be more vibrant and youthful, it's critical to learn how not to take yourself or your life too seriously, and to connect with others and reflect on the positives of your life on a regular basis. Try to do each of the following for at least fifteen minutes a day. After a week you'll really feel the beneficial effects!

Laugh It Off: Laughter is great medicine! Make an appointment to watch a TV comedy or a funny movie, or read something humorous for at least fifteen minutes a day. Sometimes you'll laugh spontaneously throughout the day, but if not, it's fine to fake it!

Connect: Take time to do something that connects you with a friend, a family member or a cause close to your heart—and by "connect," I don't mean on Facebook or on Twitter! Go retro by calling a friend on the phone, meeting up in person (perhaps to do something active) or sitting down and writing a friend or family member a good old-fashioned letter. Alternatively, you can make time to volunteer for a charitable organization, get involved at your child's school or help out at your local library. Staying connected with others and giving back are critical for your overall happiness and well-being.

Reflect: Every day think about your day and your life in a positive way. Use this time to think about what you're thankful for or to reflect on the lessons you've learned that day. A good time to do this could be after you've dropped your children off at school, during your commute or before you settle into bed. You can close your eyes and just think about, or write about, how you feel. If a negative thought enters your mind, try to reframe it into something positive and hopeful.

I Think I Can. I Think I Can. . . .

For many women, turning forty, fifty or beyond elicits positive emotions, ranging from feeling accomplished to being surprised at how quickly it all happened. But for some, celebrating another birthday, not to mention spotting a few gray hairs or seeing crow's-feet when they look in the mirror, becomes another stressor. Hormonal fluctuations and changes in your body can often make you feel lousy and perceive adverse situations as worse than they are. To help you feel empowered with each passing year, psychologist Lisa Morse, PhD, suggests the following mantras to feed to yourself often:

- I have choices. The choices I make impact how I feel.
- I am doing what is within my control to do.
- There is more to my life than X. This is only one part of me.
- No one looks at me as closely or as critically as I look at myself.
- I am as old as I think I am. Age is only a number.
- It might be a challenge, but I can do it.

VITAL SLEEP

Sleep is one of those things that can easily make or break how you feel the next day. To get the restorative, refreshing sleep you need and to set yourself up for success, aim for at least seven—and no more than nine—hours of sleep nightly. This will maximize your vitality and help your body and mind run smoothly on weekdays, weekends and even while on vacation. One way to have a more sound sleep is to eat mostly during the day, when you need the most energy, and to taper your calorie load at night (see Vitality Check: Eat By Day, Fast By Night for Better Sleep on page 204). Try this for a week, and you're bound to feel more energized and to like what you see—especially when you look in the mirror (goodbye, tired eyes). For more Stressipes to help you get just enough z's to meet your needs and not exceed them, see Chapter 11.

Eat by Day, Fast by Night for Better Sleep

Do you, like many women, tend to go hours on end without eating, skip one too many meals or consume many of your calories—if not most—after dark? Becoming a daytime eater is one of the single most important things you can do to keep your energy level in high gear and your metabolism running strong. University of Pennsylvania researcher Kelly Allison, PhD, suggests a good first step is to make it a point to eat regular meals and snacks during the day. She says, "If night eating is a pattern that has been in place for a long time, the body has come to expect food during that time, so a period of training the body that it will not receive food will be difficult, but not impossible to overcome." Karen Ansel, a registered dietitian and spokesperson for the Academy of Nutrition and Dietetics (AND), recommends the following strategies for becoming more of a daytime eater:

- **Reset your body's eating clock.** Ansel says, "Many women are so busy during the day that they hardly stop to eat anything. Then, by nighttime, they're starving. This causes a vicious cycle, because when you eat too much at night, you wake up with little, or no, appetite." She recommends capping night eating at around 8:00 p.m. and doing activities that you don't associate with eating, like reading a book, catching up on phone calls, or helping your kids with their homework or quizzing them for an upcoming test—while keeping out of the kitchen! Ansel adds, "You can also take an after-dinner walk with your family or a friend, instead of being tempted to eat in bed or in your living room while watching TV."

- **Batter up with breakfast.** Ansel recommends eating a small breakfast when you wake up, no matter how hungry you are (or aren't). She says, "It doesn't need to be much—even a simple apple with some peanut butter, a piece of whole-grain toast with hummus or a small smoothie can kick your metabolism into gear and help your body learn to front load calories."

- **Rethink your snacks.** If your kitchen is filled with far too tempting snacks, Ansel recommends seriously cleaning out your pantry and refrigerator. She says, "Once there's nothing interesting to snack on, you'll be less likely to overindulge." She recommends replacing temptations with comforting yet healthy foods, like Greek yogurt or oatmeal. "Flavored Greek yogurt, which is sweet and creamy and protein packed, is a better alternative to cookies or ice cream. It's also not the kind of thing you'd want to eat a mountain of," Ansel says. She also recommends oatmeal as a sweet and comforting evening option. "Because it's rich in complex carbohydrates, it will help your brain create serotonin to help you settle into sleep."

7-DAY VITALITY PLAN

To help you easily incorporate all the elements of the 7-Day Vitality Plan into your life, I've created a handy chart . Use this as a gentle reminder to follow the daily food, fitness and lifestyle recommendations and to stay accountable.

Daily Vitality Blueprint*

Vitality Diet**

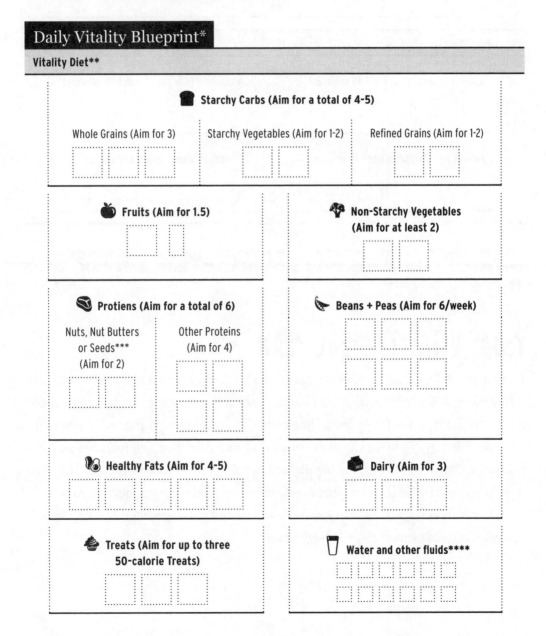

Starchy Carbs (Aim for a total of 4-5)

Whole Grains (Aim for 3)   Starchy Vegetables (Aim for 1-2)   Refined Grains (Aim for 1-2)

Fruits (Aim for 1.5)

Non-Starchy Vegetables (Aim for at least 2)

Protiens (Aim for a total of 6)

Nuts, Nut Butters or Seeds*** (Aim for 2)   Other Proteins (Aim for 4)

Beans + Peas (Aim for 6/week)

Healthy Fats (Aim for 4-5)

Dairy (Aim for 3)

Treats (Aim for up to three 50-calorie Treats)

Water and other fluids****

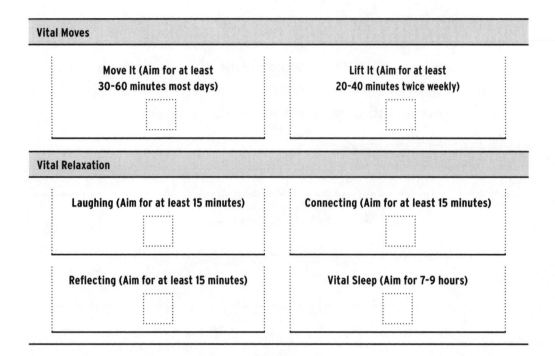

Vital Moves

Move It (Aim for at least
30-60 minutes most days)

Lift It (Aim for at least
20-40 minutes twice weekly)

Vital Relaxation

Laughing (Aim for at least 15 minutes)

Connecting (Aim for at least 15 minutes)

Reflecting (Aim for at least 15 minutes)

Vital Sleep (Aim for 7-9 hours)

*Daily goals unless otherwise noted. **These totals promote weight loss. See Appendix C for a sample template to use for weight loss or weight maintenance. ***A half an ounce nuts, nut butters or seeds each count as 1 Protein + 1 Healthy Fat. **** See Chapter 9.

7-DAY VITALITY MEAL PLAN

To keep you satisfied and to give your body the Vital Foods and nutrients it needs, the 7-Day Vitality Diet calls for three meals, one snack and even some Treats, and includes a variety of nutritious foods from the seven Vital Food groups that are convenient and user-friendly. To make the plan even easier to follow, I've also included 30 Vital Recipes in Chapter 13, which are highlighted in bold here for easy reference. This plan is designed to result in slow and steady weight loss, at a rate of about one to two pounds a week. It's also designed to help you feel satisfied and to temper food cravings, which can contribute to overeating and weight gain.

To Eat Less, "Set" Yourself Up for Success.

At home or at work, stock up on small cups, bowls, plates and serving utensils. Taking less food often means you'll eat less, and using smaller dishes to serve meals and filling them to the max will likely help you feel more satisfied with fewer calories than eating from a larger plate or bowl. Eating with smaller utensils can help you take smaller bites and fill up faster.

You can use the Vital Foods List (see page 191) to swap out items with others in the same food category if there are particular foods you don't eat or if you just want to mix things up. As for beverages, make sure to consume at least eight to nine cups of fluids (not including alcoholic beverages) throughout the day. If you consume caffeinated beverages, such as coffee or tea, do so before midday (12:00 p.m. to 2:00 p.m.) as a general rule of thumb to maximize your ability to fall asleep and stay asleep when night falls.

DAY 1

Breakfast:

1 cup shredded wheat 🍞🍞 topped with ½ medium sliced banana (½ 🍎) + 1 cup nonfat milk 🥛

Lunch:

Chopped salad made with 3 ounces cooked skinless chicken breast 🍗🍗🍗, 1 cup romaine lettuce (½ 🥦), ¼ cup plum or cherry tomatoes (¼ 🥦), ¼ cup shredded carrots (¼ 🥦) + 2 Tbs salad dressing 🥄 and 1 ounce (15) baked potato chips 🍟

Snack:

1 cup nonfat plain Greek yogurt 🥛 + trail mix made with 4 Tbs slivered almonds 🍗🍗🥄🥄, 2 Tbs dried fruit (½ 🍎) + 2 Tbs dark chocolate chips 🧁🧁

Dinner:

½ cup cooked lentils 🫛 🫛 + 1 ounce (¼ cup) shredded cheddar cheese 🧀 wrapped in one 6-inch flour tortilla 🍞, 1 cup broccoli 🥦 sautéed with 1 tsp olive oil 🥚, and ½ cup mixed berries (½ 🍎) topped with ⅓ cup whipped cream 🧁

Vital Stats: 1599 calories, 56 g fat, 17 g saturated fat, 1264 mg sodium, 115 mg cholesterol, 195mg carbohydrate, 34g fiber, 94 g protein

DAY 2

Breakfast:

½ whole wheat bagel, scooped out 🍞, topped with 2 medium slices tomato (¼ 🥦) + 1 slice melted Swiss cheese 🧀, ½ cup pineapple chunks (½ 🍎) and 1 cup nonfat milk 🥛

Lunch:

Quinoa turkey salad made with 1 cup mixed greens (½ 🥦), 2 ounces turkey breast 🍖 🍖, ½ cup mixed vegetables (carrots, cucumbers, peppers and celery) (½ 🥦), ½ cup cooked quinoa 🍞, 2 tsp olive oil 🥚🥚 + 2 Tbs balsamic vinegar and 1 cup nonfat plain yogurt 🥛

Snack:

10 cherries 🍎 + 1 ounce (14 halves) walnuts 🍖 🍖 🥚🥚

Dinner:

Beef and broccoli made with 3 ounces cooked lean beef 🍖 🍖 🍖, 1 cup broccoli 🥦 sautéed with 1 tsp oil 🥚, ½ cup brown rice 🍞, 2 steamed vegetable dumplings 🍞 (½ 🥦)+ 2 Tbs hoisin or other sauce (preferably reduced/low sodium)(70-calorie 🧁)

Vital Stats: 1575 calories, 56 g fat, 13 g saturated fat, 1704 mg sodium, 138 mg cholesterol, 182 g carbohydrate, 24 g fiber, 94 g protein

DAY 3

Breakfast:

1 slice whole-wheat toast topped with 1 Tbs peanut butter + ½ medium sliced banana (½) and 1 cup nonfat milk

Lunch:

½ panini bread filled with 1 slice (1 ounce) fresh mozzarella cheese 2 ounces grilled chicken, 1 cup red pepper strips + 1 tsp olive oil, 1 small apple, 1 cup of low-fat chocolate milk + and 12 Rold Gold pretzel twists (about 1 ounce)

Snack:

1 cup cut-up mixed veggies + 2 Tbs hummus and 3 cups **Popcorn with Mexican Topping** (see page 239)

Dinner:

3 ounces grilled turkey burger, sweet potato French fries made with 1 large sweet potato (5-6 ounces) + 1 tsp canola oil and ½ cup steamed carrots (½)

Vital Stats: 1591 calories, 50 g fat, 13 g saturated fat, 1999 mg sodium, 170 mg cholesterol, 217 g carbohydrate, 29 g fiber, 86 g protein

DAY 4

Breakfast:

1 cup cooked oatmeal mixed with ½ cup unsweetened applesauce (½) + a sprinkle of cinnamon and 1 cup nonfat milk

Lunch:

Bean salad made with 2 cups romaine lettuce, ½ cup chickpeas, ½ cup beets (½) + 3 Tbs salad dressing (1½), 1 small whole-wheat roll + 1 tsp olive oil, and 1 cup low-fat chocolate milk

Snack:

½ cup low-fat, low-sodium cottage cheese 🥛 mixed with 1 cup raspberries 🍎 and 1 ounce (about 48) pistachios 🥩 🥩 🥜 🥜

Dinner:

Pan-Seared Salmon with Mushrooms and Spinach over Sesame Brown Rice (see page 223)
🍞 (½ 🍄) (2¾ 🥩 🥩 🥩) (¾ 🥜) and 10 large (or 24 small) jelly beans 🧁 🧁

Vital Stats: 1528 calories, 53 g fat, 10 g saturated fat, 1262 mg sodium, 76 mg cholesterol, 206 g carbohydrate, 27 g fiber, 74 g protein

DAY 5

Breakfast:

1 slice whole-wheat toast 🍞 topped with 1 scrambled egg 🥩 made with nonstick cooking spray + 2 Tbs shredded cheddar cheese (½ 🥛), 1 pink grapefruit 🍎 and 1 cup nonfat milk 🥛

Lunch:

Turkey avocado pita made with 1 small whole-wheat pita 🍞 filled with 2 slices (2 ounces) turkey breast 🥩 🥩 , 2 slices romaine lettuce, 2 slices tomato (½ 🍄), 2-3 thin slices avocado 🥜 + 1 tsp mayonnaise 🥜 and 6 baby carrots (½ 🍄)

Snack:

1 cup nonfat plain Greek yogurt 🥛 topped with 2 Tbs dried fruit (½ 🍎) + 1 ounce walnuts (14 halves) 🥩 🥩 🥜 🥜

Dinner:

Vegetable pasta made with 1 cup cooked whole-wheat pasta 🍞 🍞 , 1 cup vegetables (e.g., red peppers, onions, zucchini, eggplant) 🍄 , ½ cup tofu cubes 🥩 🥩 , 2 tsp olive oil 🥜 🥜 + 2 Tbs grated Parmesan cheese (½ 🥛) and 10 large (or 24 small) jelly beans 🧁 🧁

Vital Stats: 1556 calories, 59 g fat, 12 g saturated fat, 1466 mg sodium, 245 mg cholesterol, 185 g carbohydrate, 22 g fiber, 85 g protein

DAY 6

Breakfast:

1 cup cooked oatmeal 🍞🍞 topped with 14 walnut halves 🥜🥩🥑🥑, 1 cup blueberries 🍎 and 1 cup nonfat milk 🥛

Lunch:

Tuna pita made with 1 toasted small whole-wheat pita 🍞 filled with 3 ounces tuna (½ can in water) 🥩🥩🥩 mixed with 1 tsp mayonnaise 🥑 + ½ cup chopped tomato and cucumber (½ 🥦) and 16 red grapes (½ 🍎)

Snack:

1 cup sweet peppers, baby carrots and cherry tomatoes 🥦 dipped in 2 Tbs hummus 🥩 and 1 cup nonfat milk 🥛 + 2 Oreo cookies 🧁🧁

Dinner:

Pasta with chicken made with 1 cup cooked penne pasta 🍞🍞, 3 ounces roasted skinless chicken breast 🥩🥩🥩, ½ cup tomato sauce (½ 🥦) + 2 Tbs grated Parmesan cheese (½ 🥛) and 1 cup romaine lettuce (½ 🥦) topped with 2 tsp olive oil 🥑🥑 + 2 Tbs balsamic vinegar

Vital Nutrition Stats: 1586 calories, 54 g fat, 10 g saturated fat, 1837 g sodium, 121 mg cholesterol, 190 g carbohydrate, 23 g fiber, 95 g protein

DAY 7

Breakfast:

1 cup whole-grain cereal flakes 🍞 topped with 4 Tbs slivered almonds 🥩🥩🥑🥑, 1 small orange (½ 🍎) and 1 cup nonfat milk 🥛

Lunch:

Chicken and rice bowl made with 2 ounces cooked skinless chicken breast 🥩🥩, ¼ cup black beans 🌶️, ½ cup corn 🍞, ¼ cup shredded cheddar cheese 🥛, 1 cup green peppers and tomatoes 🥦 sautéed in 1 tsp olive oil 🥑 and ½ cup cooked brown rice 🍞

Snack:

1 cup nonfat plain yogurt 🥛 topped with 4 large sliced strawberries (½ 🍎) and 1 Tbs dark chocolate chips 🧁

Dinner:

Shrimp scampi made with 3 ounces shrimp 🦐 🦐 🦐 sautéed with 1 tsp canola oil 🥑, 3 ounces (½ cup) sliced red potatoes 🍞 + 4 medium asparagus spears 🥦 roasted with 1 tsp olive oil 🥑, 2 tsp balsamic vinegar + seasonings and **Mixed Berry Delight** (see page 238) (¾ 🍎)

Vital Stats: 1600 calories, 50 g fat, 13 g saturated, 1785 mg sodium, 263 mg cholesterol, 200 g carbohydrate, 31 g fiber, 99 g protein

VITAL RECIPES

Whether you're burning the midnight oil at work; schlepping your children to school, after-school activities and weekend sports leagues; or running yourself ragged, trying to get everything crossed off your giant to-do list, it's likely that preparing healthful, wholesome and colorful meals often falls on the back burner. I'm in exactly the same car pool as you are, and I know that a busy schedule and being overextended can take their toll at mealtimes. It's extremely helpful to plan ahead to get a healthy dinner on the table in a jiffy. Fortunately, following the Vitality Diet is not a chore. In the following pages you'll find thirty Vital Recipes for breakfasts and entrées, soups, salads and sides, and snacks and desserts. Each recipe contains seven shopping ingredients or fewer (excluding pantry staples, such as spices and oils), and most take no longer than fifteen minutes to put together. You can prepare a few meals ahead of time, perhaps on a Sunday night, and freeze single-serve portions to heat and eat during the week, or when you have extra time one night to cook enough to cover you for lunch or dinner the next day. An added bonus is that all these recipes are spouse and family friendly, so everyone in your household can reap the benefits. Can't you just taste the vitality?

BREAKFASTS

BLUEBERRY BLAST

Makes five 1-cup servings.	Preparation time: 10 minutes

INGREDIENTS:

2 cups plain, nonfat yogurt

1 cup fresh blueberries

1 large frozen banana*

2 teaspoons honey

2 teaspoons ground flaxseeds

Ice, as needed

DIRECTIONS:

Combine all the ingredients in a blender and process until smooth. Use only enough ice to make the shake cold and thick, but not watery. Serve at once.

* To freeze a banana: Peel a banana, put it in a plastic ziplock bag and seal the bag. Place it in the freezer overnight, or until frozen.

Vital Stats (per serving): 109 calories, <1 g fat, <1 g saturated fat, 2 mg cholesterol, 76 mg sodium, 21 g carbohydrates, 1.7 g fiber, 16 g sugar, 6.3 g protein

ONE SERVING COUNTS AS: ($^1/_2$ 🍎), ($^1/_2$ 🥛)

BREAKFAST CITRUS FRUIT COMPOTE

Makes four $^1/_2$-cup servings.	Preparation time: 15 minutes

INGREDIENTS:

2 tangerines

1 pink grapefruit

1 navel orange

$^1/_2$ cup fresh orange juice

2 tablespoons finely minced crystallized ginger

1 tablespoon minced fresh mint

2 teaspoons honey

DIRECTIONS:

1. With a paring knife, peel the tangerines, grapefruit and orange. Separate the sections from the membranes, removing all the white pith. Place the citrus sections in a medium bowl.

2. In a small bowl, mix together the orange juice, ginger, mint and honey. Pour the orange juice mixture over the citrus sections. Let the citrus macerate for about $^1/_2$ an hour in the refrigerator.

Vital Stats (per serving): 84 calories, <1 g fat, <1 g saturated fat, 0 mg cholesterol, 2 mg sodium, 21 g carbohydrates, 2.3 g fiber, 12 g sugar, 1.2 g protein

ONE SERVING COUNTS AS: (1 🍎)

RED PEPPER AND MUSHROOM OMELET

Makes 1 serving.　　　Preparation time: 10 minutes　　　Cook time: 8 minutes

INGREDIENTS:

2 teaspoons olive oil

$\frac{1}{2}$ small red bell pepper, seeded, deribbed and diced

4 ounces sliced mixed wild mushrooms

1 clove garlic, peeled and minced

3 large egg whites

1 large egg

1 tablespoon fat-free milk

1 teaspoon salt-free Italian seasoning

$\frac{1}{4}$ teaspoon hot sauce

$\frac{1}{8}$ teaspoon freshly ground black pepper

2 tablespoons grated fresh Parmesan cheese

DIRECTIONS:

1. Heat the oil in a medium nonstick skillet over medium heat. Add the red peppers and mushrooms and sauté for about 5 minutes. Add the garlic and sauté for 1 minute.

2. Beat together the egg whites, egg, milk, Italian seasoning, hot sauce and black pepper in a small bowl. Pour the egg mixture over the vegetables. Cook for about 2 minutes, or until the eggs begin to set. Gently lift an edge of the omelet with a thin-bladed spatula and allow the uncooked eggs to flow underneath. Continue to cook for another 2 minutes, or until the omelet is almost set.

3. Sprinkle the Parmesan cheese over half the omelet and then fold the omelet in half. Reduce the heat to low and cook for 1 minute more. Slide the omelet from the pan onto a plate and serve at once.

Vital Stats (per serving): 289 calories, 17 g fat, 4.6 g saturated fat, 195 mg cholesterol, 432 mg sodium, 11 g carbohydrate, 1.3 g fiber, 4.7 g sugar, 24 g protein

ONE SERVING COUNTS AS:　(1$\frac{1}{4}$ 🥦), (2 🥩), ($\frac{1}{2}$ 🥛)

STRAWBERRY-WALNUT CINNAMON FRENCH TOAST

Makes four 1-slice servings.   Preparation time: 10 minutes   Cook time: 10 minutes

INGREDIENTS:

Butter-flavored cooking spray

1 large egg

$\frac{1}{4}$ cup fat-free milk or soy milk or almond milk

$\frac{1}{2}$ teaspoon vanilla extract

4 slices whole-grain bread

2 teaspoons non-hydrogenated buttery spread (such as Smart Balance)

1 teaspoon honey

$\frac{1}{4}$ teaspoon ground cinnamon

1 cup sliced strawberries

$\frac{1}{4}$ cup chopped toasted walnuts

DIRECTIONS:

1. Coat a large skillet with butter-flavored spray and heat it over medium heat.

2. Meanwhile, in a small shallow bowl, beat together the egg, milk and vanilla.

3. Dip a slice of the bread in the egg mixture and turn it to coat evenly. Place the bread slice in the skillet and cook on each side for 2 to 3 minutes, or until golden brown. Repeat this procedure for each slice of bread, cooking the French toast in 1 or 2 batches.

4. Mix together the buttery spread, honey and cinnamon in a 3-inch ramekin or a condiment bowl. Spread the honey-butter spread on each slice of French toast and garnish with strawberries and walnuts. Serve at once.

Vital Stats (per serving): 170 calories, 8.2 g fat, 1.8 g saturated fat, 49 mg cholesterol, 174 mg sodium, 18 g carbohydrate, 3.2 g fiber, 6 g sugar, 7 g protein

ONE SERVING COUNTS AS: (1 ■), ($\frac{1}{4}$ ●), ($\frac{3}{4}$ ◆), ($\frac{1}{2}$ ●)

WHOLE-GRAIN BLUEBERRY SCONES

Makes 6 servings.   Preparation time: 10 minutes   Cook time: 35 minutes

INGREDIENTS:

$^{1}/_{2}$ cup low-fat buttermilk

1 large egg

$1^{1}/_{4}$ cups whole-wheat pastry flour

$^{3}/_{4}$ cup unbleached all-purpose flour

2 tablespoons ground flaxseeds

2 tablespoons sugar

$1^{1}/_{2}$ teaspoons baking powder

$^{1}/_{4}$ teaspoon baking soda

$^{1}/_{4}$ teaspoon salt

3 tablespoons unsalted butter

$1^{1}/_{2}$ cups fresh blueberries

2 teaspoons grated lemon zest

DIRECTIONS:

1. Preheat the oven to 375°F. In a small bowl, mix together the buttermilk and egg, combining well.

2. In a large bowl, combine the pastry flour, all-purpose flour, flaxseeds, sugar, baking powder, baking soda and salt. With a pastry blender, cut in the butter until the mixture resembles coarse crumbs. Add the blueberries and lemon zest and mix well.

3. Make a well in the center of the dry ingredients. Add the buttermilk mixture and combine until a soft dough has formed. Add more buttermilk if needed to moisten the dough.

4. Place the dough on a lightly floured surface and knead about 4 or 5 times. Transfer the dough to an ungreased baking sheet and shape it into a 6-inch round disk. Cut the round into 6 wedges.

5. Bake for 25 minutes, or until a cake tester inserted in the center of a scone comes out clean. Remove the scones from the oven and cool them completely on a wire rack.

Vital Stats (per serving): 246 calories, 6.6 g fat, 3 g saturated fat, 39 mg cholesterol, 309 mg sodium, 42 g carbohydrate, 5.3 g fiber, 9.3 g sugar, 6.7 g protein

ONE SERVING COUNTS AS: ($1^{1}/_{2}$ 🍞), ($^{1}/_{4}$ 🍎), (50-CALORIE 🧁)

LUNCH OR DINNER ENTREES

ASIAN PEANUT CHICKEN

Makes 4 servings.   Preparation time: 15 minutes   Cook time: 15 minutes

INGREDIENTS:

1 tablespoon minced jarred ginger

1 tablespoon bottled minced garlic

2 teaspoons low-sodium soy sauce

1 teaspoon water

1 teaspoon cornstarch

$3/4$ pound chicken tenders

$1/2$ tablespoon canola oil, plus $1/2$ tablespoon for sautéing

One 8-ounce package shredded carrots

2 scallions, root ends removed and minced

$3/4$ tablespoon hoisin sauce

$1/4$ cup chopped roasted unsalted peanuts

PLAN AHEAD: 2 cups cooked whole-wheat spaghetti

DIRECTIONS:

1. In a medium bowl, combine the ginger, garlic, soy sauce, water and cornstarch. Mix well. Add the chicken tenders to the marinade and let stand for 5 minutes.

2. Heat $1/2$ tablespoon of the oil in a large wok or a large heavy skillet over high heat. Add the chicken tenders and their marinade to the skillet and stir-fry for 5 minutes. Remove the chicken from the pan and set aside.

3. Lower the heat to medium and add the remaining $1/2$ tablespoon oil to the wok or skillet. Add the carrots and scallions and stir-fry for 2 minutes. Next add the reserved chicken and stir-fry for 1 minute. Stir in the hoisin sauce, mixing well. Remove the wok or skillet from the heat and garnish the chicken with chopped peanuts. Serve the chicken over cooked whole-wheat pasta.

Vital Stats (per serving): 458 calories, 23 g fat, 4.2 g saturated fat, 38 mg cholesterol, 586 mg sodium, 44 g carbohydrate, 6.8 g fiber, 5.3 g sugar, 20 g protein

ONE SERVING COUNTS AS: (1 🍞), ($1/2$ 🥦), (3 🍖), (1 🥜), ($3/4$ 🧁)

BLACK BEAN TARTINES

Makes 4 servings.   Preparation time: 15 minutes

INGREDIENTS:

2 cups canned black beans, drained and rinsed

1 small jalapeño pepper, seeded and finely minced

2 tablespoons tomato juice (low-sodium preferred)

2 tablespoons fresh lime juice

$\frac{1}{2}$ tablespoon olive oil

2 cloves garlic, peeled and finely minced

Kosher salt or sea salt* and freshly ground black pepper, to taste

4 slices pumpernickel, rye or whole-grain bread

1 small avocado, peeled, pit removed and thinly sliced

1 small tomato, minced

DIRECTIONS:

1. Combine the black beans, jalapeño pepper, tomato juice, lime juice, olive oil, garlic, and salt and pepper in a food processor or blender, and puree until smooth but thick.

2. Spread an equal amount of the black bean puree on each of the four bread slices. Top each tartine with avocado slices and minced tomato. Serve open-faced with a fork and knife, or cut the tartines into smaller squares and eat with your hands. It doesn't get any more stress free than that!

* Not counted in Vital Stats.

Vital Stats (per serving): 249 calories, 8.2 g fat, 1.2 g saturated fat, 0 mg cholesterol, 541 mg sodium, 34 g carbohydrate, 9.7 g fiber, 3 g sugar, 10.7 g protein

ONE SERVING COUNTS AS: (1 🍞), ($\frac{1}{4}$ 🥦), (2 🐦), (1$\frac{1}{4}$ 🥑)

CARIBBEAN RED BEANS AND RICE WITH PUMPKIN SEEDS

Makes 4 servings.   Preparation time: 17 minutes   Cook time: 17 minutes

INGREDIENTS:

1 teaspoon olive oil

1 large yellow onion, peeled and diced

1 large carrot, peeled and diced

2 large cloves garlic, peeled and finely minced

Two 15-ounce cans red kidney beans, drained and rinsed

PLAN AHEAD: 2 cups cooked brown rice

2 tablespoons dry sherry

1 tablespoon balsamic vinegar

1 teaspoon dried thyme

2 bay leaves

Kosher salt* and freshly ground black pepper, to taste

$\frac{1}{4}$ cup toasted pumpkin seeds

DIRECTIONS:

1. Heat the oil in a large saucepan over medium heat. Sauté the onions, carrots and garlic for 7 to 8 minutes, or until the onions have softened.

2. Add the remaining ingredients except the pumpkin seeds. Cover and simmer on low heat for 5 minutes, or until the beans are heated through.

3. Serve hot, garnished with pumpkin seeds.

*Vital stats don't include extra sodium.

Vital Stats (per serving): 376 calories, 7 g fat, 1 g saturated fat, 0 mg cholesterol, 698 mg sodium, 62 g carbohydrates, 15 g fiber, 8 g sugar, 17 g protein

ONE SERVING COUNTS AS: (1 🍞), (1 🥦), ($\frac{3}{4}$ 🥩), (3 🐦), (1 🫘)

ITALIAN-STYLE TUNA WITH FRESH CHERRY TOMATO SAUCE

Makes 4 servings.   Preparation time: 10 minutes   Cook time: 10 minutes

INGREDIENTS:

Four 3-ounce tuna fillets

1 tablespoon salt-free garlic and herb seasoning (such as Mrs. Dash)

1 tablespoon canola oil

2 cups of cherry tomatoes, stems removed and quartered

1 tablespoon good-quality balsamic vinegar

2 tablespoons minced fresh basil

$\frac{1}{4}$ cup toasted almond slivers

1 tablespoon freshly grated Parmesan cheese

DIRECTIONS:

1. Sprinkle both sides of the tuna fillets with the garlic and herb seasoning.

2. Heat the oil in a large skillet over high heat. When the oil is hot, add the tuna and sear it for about 2 minutes on each side. Remove the tuna from the skillet to a large plate and cover with foil to keep warm.

3. Reduce the heat to medium. Add the tomatoes to the skillet and sauté for 2 minutes, or until the tomatoes are just starting to get limp. Stir in the balsamic vinegar and cook for 1 minute. Add the basil, combining well.

4. To serve, arrange the tuna fillets on individual plates. Spoon the tomato mixture evenly over each fillet, and garnish with toasted almonds and Parmesan cheese.

Vital Stats (per serving): 203 calories, 7.9 g fat, <1 g saturated fat, 41 mg cholesterol, 70 mg sodium, 5.1 g carbohydrates, 1.7 g fiber, 2.8 g sugar, 27 g protein

ONE SERVING COUNTS AS: ($\frac{1}{2}$ 🥦), (3 🐟), (1$\frac{1}{4}$ 🥜)

MEXICAN TOFU WITH MULTICOLORED PEPPERS

Makes four 1-cup servings.   Preparation time: 10 minutes   Cook time: 15 minutes

INGREDIENTS:

1 pound extra-firm tofu, cut into 1-inch cubes

2 tablespoons cornstarch, plus 1 teaspoon for sauce

$\frac{1}{4}$ teaspoon kosher salt

$\frac{1}{4}$ teaspoon freshly ground black pepper

1 tablespoon canola oil, plus 1 tablespoon for sautéing vegetables

$\frac{1}{2}$ red onion, cut into wedges

$\frac{1}{2}$ cup thinly sliced red bell pepper

$\frac{1}{2}$ cup thinly sliced yellow bell pepper

$\frac{1}{2}$ cup thinly sliced green bell pepper

$\frac{1}{2}$ small jalapeño pepper, seeded and minced

$\frac{1}{3}$ cup low-fat, reduced-sodium chicken broth

$\frac{1}{4}$ cup minced cilantro

DIRECTIONS:

1. Place the tofu in a large bowl. Sprinkle the tofu with the 2 tablespoons cornstarch, salt and pepper. Toss to coat.

2. Heat 1 tablespoon of the oil in a large wok or a heavy pan over medium-high heat. Add the tofu, in batches if necessary, and cook for 3 minutes, browning it on all sides. Remove the tofu from the pan to a large plate and keep warm.

3. Add the remaining 1 tablespoon oil to the pan, and then add the onions and stir-fry for 2 minutes. Add the bell peppers and jalapeño pepper and stir-fry for 2 minutes.

4. In a small bowl, mix together the chicken broth and the remaining 1 teaspoon cornstarch. Pour the broth over the peppers and onions and stir to coat. Return the tofu to the pan and then add the cilantro. Toss and serve at once.

Vital Stats (per serving): 194 calories, 12 g fat, 1.1 g saturated fat, 0 mg cholesterol, 226 mg sodium, 12 g carbohydrates, 1.8 g fiber, 2.3 g sugar, 10.3 g protein

ONE SERVING COUNTS AS: ($\frac{1}{2}$ 🥦), (2 🍖), (1$\frac{1}{2}$ 🫘)

PAN-SEARED SALMON WITH MUSHROOMS AND SPINACH OVER SESAME BROWN RICE

Makes 4 servings.　　Preparation time: 15 minutes　　Cook time: 15 minutes

INGREDIENTS:

1 teaspoon olive or canola oil, plus 1 teaspoon for sautéing vegetables

Four 3-ounce salmon fillets

Kosher salt* and freshly ground black pepper, to taste

1 tablespoon minced shallots

1$\frac{1}{2}$ cups presliced mushrooms

2 cups fresh baby spinach

1 teaspoon grated lemon zest

1 teaspoon fresh lemon juice

PLAN AHEAD: 2 cups cooked brown rice**

2 tablespoons toasted sesame seeds

DIRECTIONS:

1. Heat 1 teaspoon of the oil in a large skillet over medium-high heat. Sprinkle the salmon fillets lightly with salt and pepper. Add the salmon to the skillet and sear for about 5 minutes on each side, or until the salmon is cooked through. Remove the salmon from the skillet to a large plate and cover with foil to keep warm.

2. Add the remaining 1 teaspoon oil to the skillet. Add the shallots and sauté for 1 minute. Place the mushrooms in the skillet in a single layer and sauté for 2 minutes without stirring. Then stir the mushrooms and cook for 2 minutes more. Add the spinach and cook for 30 seconds, or until the spinach wilts. Remove the skillet from the heat and stir in the lemon zest and lemon juice.

3. Mix together the brown rice and sesame seeds. Spoon the rice onto individual plates and top with the mushroom-spinach mixture. Arrange a salmon fillet atop each bed of rice.

* Vital stats don't include extra sodium. **Vital Tip: Cooking brown rice from scratch can take 40 minutes. Use precooked packages (such as Uncle Ben's) from your local grocery store instead to save time and stress less.

Vital Stats (per serving): 285 calories, 10.6 g fat, 1.6 g saturated fat, 47 mg cholesterol, 58 mg sodium, 26 g carbohydrate, 3.3 g fiber, 1.4 g sugar, 22 g protein

ONE SERVING COUNTS AS: (1 🍞), ($\frac{1}{2}$ 🥦), (2$\frac{3}{4}$ 🥩), ($\frac{3}{4}$ 🥜)

SEARED HALIBUT WITH WALNUT SPINACH

Makes 4 servings.　　Preparation time: 5 minutes　　Cook time: 13 minutes

INGREDIENTS:

2 teaspoons olive oil

1 pound halibut fillets, about $\frac{1}{2}$ inch-thick, patted really dry

$\frac{1}{2}$ teaspoon kosher salt

$\frac{1}{2}$ teaspoon lemon-pepper seasoning

$\frac{1}{4}$ cup dry white wine or reduced-sodium, low-fat chicken broth

1 medium shallot, peeled and minced

$1\frac{1}{2}$ pounds fresh baby spinach leaves

$\frac{1}{4}$ cup chopped toasted walnuts

$\frac{1}{8}$ teaspoon crushed red pepper flakes

1 tablespoon fresh lemon zest

DIRECTIONS:

1. Heat the olive oil in a large skillet over medium-high heat. Sprinkle the halibut fillets with salt and lemon-pepper seasoning. Place the fillets in the skillet and sear for 4 to 5 minutes on each side, or until golden brown. Remove the halibut fillets from the skillet to a large plate. Tent with foil to keep warm.

2. Add the wine or broth to the skillet, scraping up any browned bits, and cook for 30 seconds. Add the shallots to the skillet and sauté for 2 minutes. Next add the spinach and, using a pair of tongs, turn the spinach until it just wilts, not allowing it to release much liquid. Add the walnuts and red pepper flakes and toss.

3. Place the spinach on individual plates and arrange the halibut atop the spinach. Sprinkle with fresh lemon zest and serve at once.

Vital Stats (per serving): 321 calories, 23 g fat, 3.6 g saturated fat, 52 mg cholesterol, 539 mg sodium, 8 g carbohydrate, 4.5 g fiber, 1 g sugar, 22 g protein

ONE SERVING COUNTS AS:　　(1 🥦), (3 🍖), ($\frac{1}{2}$ 🥜)

SHRIMP AND BROCCOLI BOWL

Makes 4 servings.   Preparation time: 5 minutes   Cook time: 12 minutes

INGREDIENTS:

12 ounces large shrimp, peeled and deveined

4 cloves garlic, peeled and minced

1 teaspoon salt-free Italian seasoning

$\frac{1}{4}$ teaspoon crushed red pepper flakes

$\frac{1}{2}$ tablespoon olive oil, plus $\frac{1}{2}$ tablespoon for sautéing vegetables

$\frac{1}{2}$ cup minced onion

2 cups broccoli florets

$\frac{1}{2}$ medium red bell pepper, seeded, deribbed and thinly sliced

$\frac{1}{4}$ cup water

1 tablespoon fresh lemon juice

$\frac{1}{4}$ teaspoon freshly ground black pepper

PLAN AHEAD: 2 cups frozen brown rice, cooked according to package directions (optional)

DIRECTIONS:

1. In a medium bowl, combine the shrimp, garlic, Italian seasoning and red pepper flakes.

2. Heat the $\frac{1}{2}$ tablespoon olive oil in a large skillet over medium-high heat. Add the shrimp and sauté for 2 to 3 minutes, or until cooked through. Remove the shrimp from the skillet to a plate and set aside.

3. Add the remaining $\frac{1}{2}$ tablespoon oil to the skillet. Add the onions and sauté for 3 minutes. Add the broccoli and sauté for 2 minutes. Then add the red peppers and sauté for 1 minute. Pour in the water, cover and steam for 2 minutes, or until the broccoli is bright green. Season the vegetables with lemon juice and black pepper. Return the shrimp to the skillet and stir.

4. Serve the shrimp and broccoli over brown rice, if desired.

Vital Stats (per serving): 231 calories, 5.4 g fat, <1 g saturated fat, 107 mg cholesterol, 503 mg sodium, 30 g carbohydrate, 3.5 g fiber, 3 g sugar, 16 g protein

ONE SERVING COUNTS AS: (1 🍞), (1 🥦), (3 🍖)

TOFU SANDWICHES

Makes 4 servings.   Preparation time: 15 minutes   Cook time: 7 minutes

INGREDIENTS:

1 pound extra-firm, water-packed tofu

1 tablespoon canola oil

$\frac{1}{2}$ cup prepared barbecue sauce (reduced sugar/sodium)

$1\frac{1}{2}$ cups prepared coleslaw mix

2 tablespoons reduced-fat mayonnaise

2 teaspoons apple cider vinegar

Salt* and freshly ground black pepper, to taste

4 whole-wheat hamburger buns, toasted

4 tomato slices

DIRECTIONS:

1. Drain the block of tofu. Wrap the tofu in two layers of paper towels. Press down slightly to remove the excess water. Remove the paper towels and discard.

2. Stand the tofu on its long, more narrow end and cut lengthwise into 4 rectangles about $\frac{1}{2}$-inch thick.

3. Heat the oil in a large nonstick skillet. Add the tofu and cook until it is browned on both sides, about 4 minutes per side. Add the barbecue sauce and turn the tofu to coat it with the sauce. Cover and cook for 1 minute.

4. Meanwhile, mix together the coleslaw mix, mayonnaise and vinegar and then season the coleslaw with salt and pepper.

5. Spoon some coleslaw on the bottom of each hamburger bun. Place a tofu rectangle and a tomato slice on each one, and then arrange the hamburger bun tops on top.

*Vital stats don't include extra sodium.

Vital Stats (per serving): 343 calories, 14 g fat, 1.8 g saturated fat, 3 mg cholesterol, 494 mg sodium, 40 g carbohydrate, 5.6 g fiber, 15 g sugar, 16 g protein

ONE SERVING COUNTS AS: (1 🍞), ($\frac{1}{2}$ 🥦), (2 🍶), (1 🧆)

SOUPS, SALADS AND SIDES

ASIAN BROCCOLI SALAD

Makes four 1-cup servings.　　Preparation time: 15 minutes　　Cook time: 10-15 minutes

INGREDIENTS:

1$\frac{1}{2}$ pounds broccoli

2 scallions, root ends removed and minced

2 cloves garlic, peeled and minced

2 tablespoons low-sodium soy sauce

2 tablespoon rice vinegar

1 tablespoon peanut oil

$\frac{1}{2}$ teaspoon toasted sesame oil

DIRECTIONS:

1. Fill a 4-quart saucepan two-thirds full with water, and bring it to a boil over medium-high heat. Meanwhile, peel the broccoli stalks and slice them into thin pieces. Cut the florets into bite-size pieces. Add the broccoli to the boiling water, turn off the heat and let the broccoli stand in the hot water for 3 minutes. Drain and rinse the broccoli in cold water and drain again.

2. Mix together the scallions, garlic, soy sauce, vinegar, peanut oil and sesame oil in a large serving bowl. Add the broccoli and toss to coat. Cover and refrigerate the salad for 1 to 2 hours prior to serving.

Vital Stats (per serving): 108 calories, 4.7 g fat, 0.8 g saturated fat, 0 mg cholesterol, 338 mg sodium, 15 g carbohydrate, 5.9 g fiber, 3.7 g sugar, 4.7 g protein

ONE SERVING COUNTS AS:　　(1$\frac{1}{2}$ 🥦), (1 🫙)

BEET AND CARROT SALAD

Makes four 1-cup servings. Preparation time: 25 minutes

INGREDIENTS:

Salad:

2 large beets, peeled

2 large carrots, peeled

$\frac{1}{4}$ cup toasted walnut pieces

1 large shallot, minced

2 tablespoons minced fresh chives

Dressing:

3 tablespoons rice vinegar

1 clove garlic, peeled and minced

1 teaspoon Dijon mustard

2 tablespoons peanut* or canola oil

Salt** and freshly ground black pepper, to taste

DIRECTIONS:

1. Using a handheld box grater or the shred blade on a food processor, shred the beets and carrots. Place the shredded beets and carrots, walnuts, shallots and chives in a large bowl and mix well.

2. In a small bowl, mix together the rice vinegar, garlic and mustard. Slowly add the oil in a thin stream and whisk until it has emulsified. Season the dressing with salt and pepper and then pour it over the beet-carrot mixture and mix well.

* Analysis used peanut oil. **Vital stats don't include extra sodium.

Vital Stats (per serving): 152 calories, 11 g fat, 1.6 g saturated fat, 0 mg cholesterol, 74 mg sodium, 12 g carbohydrate, 3.1 g fiber, 7 g sugar, 2.4 g protein

ONE SERVING COUNTS AS: ($\frac{1}{2}$ 🥦), ($\frac{1}{2}$ 🍵), (2 🥜)

EDAMAME AND WILD RICE SALAD WITH FLAXSEEDS

Makes six 1-cup servings.   Preparation time: 10 minutes

INGREDIENTS:

Salad:

PLAN AHEAD: 2 cups shelled edamame, cooked according to package directions, cooled to room temperature

PLAN AHEAD: 1 cup cooked wild rice

1 large carrot, peeled and diced

$\frac{1}{2}$ cup minced red onion

$\frac{1}{2}$ cup minced celery

1 cup halved cherry tomatoes

3 tablespoons dry-roasted* flaxseedss

Dressing:

2 tablespoons fresh lemon juice

1 teaspoon Dijon mustard

$\frac{1}{2}$ teaspoon sugar

1 clove garlic, peeled and finely minced

$\frac{1}{4}$ cup olive oil

$\frac{1}{4}$ teaspoon kosher salt

$\frac{1}{4}$ teaspoon freshly ground black pepper

Six romaine lettuce leaves

DIRECTIONS:

1. In a large bowl, combine the edamame, wild rice, carrots, red onions and celery and mix well. Fold in the cherry tomatoes and flaxseedss and set aside.

2. In a small bowl, whisk together the lemon juice, mustard, sugar and garlic. Slowly add the olive oil in a thin stream and whisk until the dressing has emulsified. Season with salt and pepper.

3. Pour the dressing over the edamame-rice mixture and mix well. Line a platter with the romaine lettuce leaves, spoon the salad on top and serve at once.

* You can also buy whole flaxseedss, grind them, add them to a dry skillet and toast over medium heat for 2 to 3 minutes.

Vital Stats (per serving): 190 calories, 12.6 g fat, 1.4 g saturated fat, 0 mg cholesterol, 112 mg sodium, 15 g carbohydrate, 4.5 g fiber, 3.7 g sugar, 6.4 g protein

ONE SERVING COUNTS AS: ($\frac{1}{2}$ 🥦), ($1\frac{1}{2}$ 🍲), ($2\frac{1}{4}$ 🫘)

ITALIAN BEANS AND GREENS

Makes four 1-cup servings.   Preparation time: 10 minutes   Cook time: 12 minutes

INGREDIENTS:

1 tablespoon olive oil

1 small onion, peeled and diced

3 cloves garlic, peeled and minced

4 cups torn kale leaves (ribs removed)

$\frac{1}{4}$ cup low-fat, low-sodium chicken broth

3 cups canned chickpeas (drained and rinsed)

One 14$\frac{1}{2}$-ounce can Italian-style diced tomatoes (no salt added), drained

1 teaspoon sugar

$\frac{1}{2}$ teaspoon dried oregano

$\frac{1}{2}$ teaspoon dried basil

$\frac{1}{2}$ teaspoon kosher salt

$\frac{1}{4}$ teaspoon freshly ground black pepper

DIRECTIONS:

1. Heat the oil in a large skillet over medium heat. Add the onions and garlic and sauté for 3 minutes. Next add the kale and sauté for 3 minutes. Pour in the broth, cover and steam the vegetables for 2 to 3 minutes.

2. Uncover the skillet and add the chickpeas, tomatoes, sugar, oregano, basil, salt and pepper. Cover and cook for 5 minutes, or until all the chickpeas are heated through.

Vital Stats (per serving): 271 calories, 6.9 g fat, 0.8 g saturated fat, 0 mg cholesterol, 539 mg sodium, 43 g carbohydrate, 4.8 g fiber, 6 g sugar, 12 g protein

ONE SERVING COUNTS AS: (1$\frac{1}{2}$ 🥦), (3 🐦), ($\frac{3}{4}$ 🥚)

KALE AND BLUEBERRY SALAD

Makes four 1-cup servings. Preparation time: 15 minutes

INGREDIENTS:

Salad:

3 cups finely chopped kale leaves (ribs removed)

$^2/_3$ cup fresh blueberries

$^1/_4$ cup toasted walnuts

$^1/_4$ cup very finely minced shallots

Dressing:

2 tablespoons fresh lemon juice

1 tablespoon white wine vinegar

1 clove garlic, peeled and finely minced

$^1/_2$ teaspoon sugar

2 tablespoons walnut oil

DIRECTIONS:

1. Combine the kale, blueberries, walnuts and shallots in a large bowl.

2. In a small bowl, whisk together the lemon juice, white wine vinegar, garlic and sugar. Slowly add the oil in a thin stream and whisk until the dressing has emulsified.

3. Add the dressing to the kale-blueberry mixture and toss well, using tongs.

4. Arrange the salad on individual plates and serve at once.

Vital Stats (per serving): 154 calories, 11.4 g fat, 1 g saturated fat, 0 mg cholesterol, 24 mg sodium, 13 g carbohydrate, 3.3 g fiber, 5.3 g sugar, 3.3 g protein

ONE SERVING COUNTS AS: ($^1/_2$ 🥦), ($^1/_2$ 🫐), (2 🥜)

ROMAINE SALAD WITH RASPBERRIES

Makes seven 1-cup servings.   Preparation time: 20 minutes

INGREDIENTS:

Dressing:

1 cup fresh raspberries

2 tablespoons fresh lemon juice

1 tablespoon honey

$\frac{1}{2}$ teaspoon Dijon mustard

$\frac{1}{4}$ cup olive oil

$\frac{1}{4}$ teaspoon kosher salt

$\frac{1}{4}$ teaspoon freshly ground black pepper

Salad:

5 cups torn romaine lettuce leaves

$\frac{1}{2}$ medium red onion, peeled and thinly sliced

1 small red bell pepper, seeded, deribbed and thinly sliced

1 cup fresh raspberries

$\frac{1}{4}$ cup toasted walnuts

DIRECTIONS:

1. Prepare the dressing by placing the raspberries in a fine sieve over a small bowl to catch the juice. Using a fork, mash the raspberries to extract their juice. Discard the pulp. Add the lemon juice, honey and mustard to the raspberry juice and whisk. Slowly add the olive oil in a thin stream, whisking constantly until the dressing has emulsified. Stir in the salt and pepper, and set the dressing aside.

2. Place the romaine lettuce, onions and bell peppers in a large bowl. Add the whole raspberries and the dressing and toss gently.

3. Spoon the salad onto individual plates and garnish with walnuts. Serve at once.

Vital Stats (per serving): 132 calories, 10.4 g fat, 1.3 g saturated fat, 0 mg cholesterol, 77 mg sodium, 10 g carbohydrate, 3.6 g fiber, 5.3 g sugar, 1.6 g protein

ONE SERVING COUNTS AS: ($\frac{1}{4}$ 🍎), ($\frac{1}{2}$ 🥦), ($\frac{1}{2}$ 🥜), (2 🫒)

SHREDDED BRUSSELS SPROUTS

Makes five 1-cup servings.　　Preparation time: 20 minutes　　Cook time: 8-12 minutes

INGREDIENTS:

1 pound (about 5 cups) fresh small Brussels sprouts

2 teaspoons olive oil

$\frac{1}{2}$ cup diced onion

2 teaspoons fresh lemon juice

1 teaspoon fresh lemon zest

Kosher salt*, freshly ground black pepper or minced garlic, to taste

DIRECTIONS:

1. Trim the hard ends off the Brussels sprouts. Remove any outer leaves that have yellowed or withered. Cut each Brussels sprout in half and then slice the halves into thin strips. Set aside.

2. Heat the oil in a large skillet over medium-high heat. Add the onions and sauté for 3 to 4 minutes, or until they have softened. Add the Brussels sprouts and toss, using tongs, to coat them with the onions. Cook for about 5 to 7 minutes, or until the Brussels sprouts have browned.

3. Sprinkle the Brussels sprouts with the lemon juice and lemon zest. Season with salt and pepper, if desired.

* Not counted in Vital Stats.

Vital Stats (per serving): 58 calories, 2.3 g fat, 0.4 g saturated fat, 0 mg cholesterol, 20 mg sodium, 8.8 g carbohydrate, 2.7 g fiber, 2.6 g sugar, 2.6 g protein

ONE SERVING COUNTS AS:　　(1 🥦), ($\frac{1}{2}$ 🫒)

TUSCAN SOUP WITH SPINACH AND SWEET POTATO

Makes eight 1-cup servings.   Preparation time: 15 minutes   Cook time: 25-30 minutes

INGREDIENTS:

1 tablespoon olive oil

$\frac{1}{2}$ cup diced onion

2 cloves garlic, peeled and minced

1 large sweet potato, peeled and cut into $\frac{1}{2}$-inch dice

1 teaspoon dried basil

1 teaspoon dried oregano

Pinch of crushed red pepper flakes

4 cups low-fat, low-sodium chicken broth

One 14$\frac{1}{2}$-ounce can diced Italian-style tomatoes (no salt added)

2 cups baby spinach leaves

1 cup canned chickpeas (drained and rinsed)

DIRECTIONS:

1. Heat the oil in a large saucepan over medium heat. Add the onions and garlic, and sauté for 3 to 4 minutes, or until the onions have softened. Next add the sweet potatoes and sauté for 5 minutes.

2. Add the basil, oregano and red pepper flakes to the saucepan, and sauté for 2 minutes. Stir in the broth and tomatoes and bring to a boil. Lower the heat and simmer for 10 minutes, uncovered.

3. Add the spinach and chickpeas and cook until the spinach wilts, about 2 to 3 minutes. Taste and adjust the seasoning.

Vital Stats (per serving): 93 calories, 3 g fat, 0.5 g saturated fat, 0 mg cholesterol, 94 mg sodium, 12.7 g carbohydrate, 1.3 g fiber, 3.2 g sugar, 4.8 g protein

ONE SERVING COUNTS AS: ($\frac{1}{4}$ 🍞), ($\frac{1}{4}$ 🥦), ($\frac{1}{2}$ 🐦), ($\frac{1}{2}$ 🫘)

WHITE BEAN AND KALE SOUP

Makes seven 1-cup servings.   Preparation time: 15 minutes   Cook time: 15 minutes

INGREDIENTS:

2 teaspoons olive oil

1 large onion, peeled and diced

1 large carrot, peeled and diced

2 celery stalks, diced

2 cloves garlic, peeled and minced

2 teaspoons dried rosemary

Two 15-ounce cans chickpeas, drained and rinsed

$3\frac{1}{2}$ cups low-fat, low-sodium chicken broth

One $14\frac{1}{2}$-ounce can diced tomatoes (no salt added)

2 cups minced kale leaves (ribs removed)

Salt* and freshly ground black pepper, to taste

DIRECTIONS:

1. Heat the oil in a large pot over medium heat. Reduce the heat to medium-low, add the onions, carrots and celery and sauté for 6 to 7 minutes. Next add the garlic and rosemary and sauté for 1 minute.

2. Stir in the chickpeas, broth and tomatoes and bring to a boil. Lower the heat and simmer for 10 minutes. Add the kale and simmer for 5 minutes more. Season with salt and pepper.

* Vital stats don't include extra sodium.

Vital Stats (per serving): 239 calories, 5.3 g fat, 0.7 g saturated fat, 0 mg cholesterol, 326 mg sodium, 38 g carbohydrate, 2.2 g fiber, 4 g sugar, 12.6 g protein

ONE SERVING COUNTS AS: (1 🥦), (2 🐦)

SNACKS AND DESSERTS

BLUEBERRIES WITH RICOTTA CREAM

Makes four ¹/₂-cup servings. Preparation time: 5 minutes

INGREDIENTS:

2 cups fresh blueberries

2 tablespoons sugar

2 tablespoons fresh
lime juice

¹/₂ cup part-skim ricotta
cheese

¹/₄ cup plain nonfat
Greek yogurt

¹/₂ teaspoon lime zest

DIRECTIONS:

1. In a medium bowl, combine the blueberries, sugar and
    lime juice. Cover and refrigerate.
2. Mix together the ricotta cheese, yogurt and lime zest
    in a small bowl. Serve the blueberries with a dollop of
    the ricotta cream.

Vital Stats (per serving): 119 calories, 2.7 g fat, 1.6 g saturated fat, 10 mg cholesterol, 45 mg sodium, 20 g carbohydrate, 1.8 g fiber, 14.4 g sugar, 5.4 g protein

ONE SERVING COUNTS AS: (¹/₂ 🍎), (¹/₃ 🧀)

CHERRY YOGURT SUNDAES

Makes 4 servings. Preparation time: 10 minutes Cook time: 2 minutes

INGREDIENTS:

1 pound (2 cups) fresh or
frozen (thawed) pitted cherries, coarsely chopped

¹/₂ cup cherry jam
(no sugar added)

1 tablespoon water

2 teaspoons cornstarch

2 cups nonfat vanilla yogurt

¹/₄ cup toasted walnuts

DIRECTIONS:

1. Combine the cherries and jam in a large saucepan.
    Mix together the water and cornstarch in a cup until
    smooth. Stir the cornstarch mixture into the cherries.
    Bring to a simmer over medium heat and cook for
    about 1 minute, or until thickened.
2. Spoon the yogurt into dessert bowls. Top with the
    warm cherry sauce, garnish with walnuts and serve
    at once.

Vital Stats (per serving): 305 calories, 4 g fat, 0.4 g saturated fat, 3 mg cholesterol, 90 mg sodium, 59 g carbohydrate, 1.2 g fiber, 56 g sugar, 8.6 g protein

ONE SERVING COUNTS AS: (1 🍎), (¹/₂ 🍬), (¹/₂ 🥜), (¹/₂ 🧀), (40-CALORIE 🧁)

CHOCOLATE WALNUT GRANOLA BARS

Makes 21 servings.   Preparation time: 10 minutes   Cook time: 10-15 minutes

INGREDIENTS:

2 cups rolled oats (not quick cooking)

1 cup coarsely chopped walnuts

1 cup sunflower seeds

$^3/_4$ cup wheat germ

$^2/_3$ cup brown sugar

$^1/_2$ cup honey or light agave nectar

2 tablespoons unsalted butter or non-hydrogenated buttery spread (such as Smart Balance)

$^1/_2$ teaspoon vanilla extract

$^1/_3$ cup dark chocolate chips or chunks

DIRECTIONS:

1. Preheat the oven to 375°F. Line a 9 x 13-inch baking pan with waxed paper with 3 inches on two ends of the pan as overhang.

2. In a large bowl, combine the oats, walnuts, sunflower seeds and wheat germ. Spread the mixture on two large ungreased baking sheets and toast in the oven for about 10 minutes, stirring occasionally to prevent burning. Set aside.

3. Combine the brown sugar, honey or agave nectar, butter or spread and vanilla in a small saucepan. Cook over medium heat until the brown sugar melts and the mixture is liquidy.

4. Transfer the reserved oat-walnut mixture to a large bowl. Pour the brown sugar mixture over the oat-walnut mixture and combine well. Fold in the chocolate chips.

5. Spoon the granola mixture into the waxed paper-lined baking pan and spread it out evenly with a wooden spoon. Fold the excess waxed paper on each end over the top of the granola mixture. Place another sheet of waxed paper on top of the granola mixture, covering it, and press down slightly. Let the granola mixture cool on the counter for 1 to 2 hours.

6. Remove the top sheet of waxed paper. Lift the granola rectangle out of the pan by holding on to the excess waxed paper on each end, and transfer it to a large plate. With a sharp knife, cut the granola into 3 x 1$^1/_2$-inch bars. Store the granola bars in an airtight container for about a week.

Vital Stats (per serving): 194 calories, 9.8 g fat, 2.1 g saturated fat, 3 mg cholesterol, 4.5 mg sodium, 25 g carbohydrate, 2.5 g fiber, 15.6 g sugar, 4.3 g protein

ONE SERVING COUNTS AS: ($^1/_2$ 🍞), (1 🥜), (1 🥜), (50-CALORIE 🧁)

MIXED BERRY DELIGHT

Makes eight $\frac{1}{2}$-cup servings.　　　Preparation time: 10 minutes

INGREDIENTS:

1 cup sliced fresh strawberries, plus 1 cup for mixing with other berries

$\frac{1}{3}$ cup white grape juice

1 tablespoon honey

$\frac{1}{2}$ cup nonfat vanilla yogurt

2 cups fresh berries (blueberries,* raspberries and/or blackberries)

DIRECTIONS:

1.　In a blender, combine the 1 cup strawberries, grape juice and honey and puree.

2.　Pour the puree into a medium bowl. Fold in the remaining strawberries and the yogurt.

3.　Place the mixed berries in dessert bowls or ramekins. Spoon the strawberry sauce over the mixed berries and serve at once.

* Used for nutritional analysis.

Vital Stats (per serving): 61 calories, <1 g fat, 0 g saturated fat, 0 mg cholesterol, 13 mg sodium, 14.5 g carbohydrate, 1.7 g fiber, 11.6 g sugar, 1.3 g protein

ONE SERVING COUNTS AS: ($\frac{3}{4}$ 🍎)

POPCORN (AND TOPPERS)

Makes about five 3-cup servings.   Preparation time: 5-10 minutes

INGREDIENTS:

"Fake" cheese topping:

2-3 tablespoons nutritional yeast

$\frac{1}{2}$ teaspoon salt

Cinnamon topping:

2 teaspoons ground cinnamon

2 teaspoons sugar

Mexican topping:

2 teaspoons mild or hot chili powder

$\frac{1}{2}$ teaspoon ground cumin

$\frac{1}{2}$ teaspoon dried oregano

$\frac{1}{2}$ teaspoon salt

Popcorn:

$\frac{1}{2}$ cup unpopped corn

1 tablespoon olive oil

Olive oil-flavored or butter-flavored cooking spray, to coat popcorn

DIRECTIONS:

1. Prepare each of the toppings by mixing together the ingredients for each in a small bowl. Set aside.

2. Air pop the popcorn to yield about 3 quarts popcorn. Alternatively, add 1 tablespoon olive oil to a large pot and place 2 kernels of popcorn in it. Heat the oil over medium-high heat. When the kernels in the pot pop, add the rest of the popcorn and cover. Pop the popcorn, shaking the pot several times to ensure even cooking.

3. Pour the popcorn into a large bowl. Lightly coat the popcorn with the cooking spray. Sprinkle on the topping of choice and toss the popcorn. Serve at once.

For Popcorn with "Fake" Cheese Topping:
Vital Stats (per serving): 123 calories, 4 g fat, 0.5 g saturated fat, 0 mg cholesterol, 119 mg sodium, 18 g carbohydrate, 3.9 g fiber, 0 g sugar, 4.5 g protein

ONE SERVING COUNTS AS: (1 🍞), (1 🥜)

For Popcorn with Cinnamon Topping:
Vital Stats (per serving): 119 calories, 3.8 g fat, 0.5 g saturated fat, 0 mg cholesterol, 2 mg sodium, 19.3 g carbohydrate, 3.4 g fiber, 1.9 g sugar, 2.5 g protein

ONE SERVING COUNTS AS: (1 🍞), (1 🥜)

For Popcorn with Mexican Topping:
Vital Stats (per serving): 114 calories, 4 g fat, 0.6 g saturated fat, 0 mg cholesterol, 136 mg sodium, 17.5 g carbohydrate, 3.4 g fiber, 0 g sugar, 2.7 g protein

ONE SERVING COUNTS AS: (1 🍞), (1 🥜)

SPICY EDAMAME

Makes four ¹/₂-cup servings.   Preparation time: 5 minutes   Cook time: 15 minutes

INGREDIENTS:

One 10-ounce package shelled edamame (thawed and patted dry)

2 teaspoons canola oil

1 tablespoon Southwestern seasoning blend (such as Mrs. Dash)

DIRECTIONS:

1. Preheat the oven to 400°F. Line a baking sheet with parchment paper.

2. In a large bowl, mix together the edamame, oil and seasoning.

3. Spread the edamame in a single layer on the prepared baking sheet. Bake the edamame for about 15 minutes, or until golden brown. Transfer the edamame to a medium bowl and serve at once.

Vital Stats (per serving): 99 calories, 5.7 g fat, 0.2 g saturated fat, 0 mg cholesterol, 4 mg sodium, 6 g carbohydrate, 3.4 g fiber, 1.8 g sugar, 7.3 g protein

ONE SERVING COUNTS AS: (2¹/₂ 🫘), (¹/₂ 🥜)

STRAWBERRY AQUA FRESCA

Makes four 1-cup servings.   Preparation time: 5 minutes

INGREDIENTS:

2¹/₂ cups coarsely chopped fresh strawberries

3 tablespoons sugar

2 tablespoons fresh lime juice

2 cups cold water

Ice

DIRECTIONS:

1. In a blender, puree the strawberries. Add the sugar and lime juice and process for 1 minute.

2. Pour the strawberry puree into a pitcher. Stir in the water, mixing well. Cover and refrigerate until cold, about 2 hours. Serve over ice in tall glasses.

Vital Stats (per serving): 72 calories, < 1 g fat, 0 g saturated fat, 0 mg cholesterol, 6 mg sodium, 18 g carbohydrate, 2.1 g fiber, 14.7 g sugar, 0.7 g protein

ONE SERVING COUNTS AS: (³/₄ 🍎)

VITALITY MENU IDEAS

To help you incorporate the Vitality Diet into your life—not just for seven days, but for a lifetime—I've created a flexible mix-and-match menu with breakfasts, lunches, dinners and snacks. You'll also find a few more of the Vital Recipes that appear in Chapter 13 highlighted here for easy reference. Whether you're eating out or on the go or simply want a little more choice and flexibility, these options are sure to satisfy. Each meal provides an average of 450 calories, and each snack provides an average of 200 calories. If you choose one option for each meal and snack daily, you can top those off with one 50-calorie treat (see the Treat Cheat Sheet on page 199). Use the Vital Foods List in Chapter 12 to easily swap out any Vital Foods or Treats listed with a similar option.

BREAKFAST

OPTION 1

1 cup shredded wheat topped with ½ ounce (7 halves) walnuts + 1 cup nonfat milk + 1 cup mixed berries

OPTION 2

1 cup cooked oatmeal topped with 1 cup sliced strawberries + 1 cup nonfat milk, and 1 deviled egg made with 1 hard-boiled egg + 1 tsp mayonnaise + a sprinkle of paprika

OPTION 3 (1⅔) (½) (½)

Breakfast burrito made with 1 small whole-wheat flour tortilla, 1 whole egg, 2 egg whites, 2 Tbs shredded cheddar cheese, ½ cup tomatoes + non-stick cooking spray + 1 cup mixed berries

OPTION 4 (1¼) (½)

Red Pepper and Mushroom Omelet (see page 215) + 1 slice whole-wheat bread, toasted and topped with 1 tsp vegetable oil spread + ½ cup pineapple + ½ cup nonfat milk

OPTION 5 (½)

1 whole-wheat English muffin, toasted, topped with 1 Tbs almond butter + 1 cup nonfat Greek yogurt, mixed with 2 Tbs dried fruit

OPTION 6 (¼)

½ bagel topped with 1 slice turkey breast, 1 slice tomato and 1 slice muenster cheese, melted + **Breakfast Citrus Fruit Compote (see page 214)**

OPTION 7

1 cup nonfat Greek yogurt topped with 1 ounce almonds (24 whole or 4 Tbs chopped) and 1 cup mixed berries

LUNCH

OPTION 1 (1½) (1½)

White Bean and Kale Soup (see page 235) + mozzarella and tomato salad made with 1½ ounces mozzarella cheese, 3-4 slices tomato, 1 tsp olive oil and 1-2 Tbs balsamic vinegar

OPTION 2 (¼) (½) (3½)

Romaine Salad with Raspberries (see page 232) + chicken sandwich made with 3 ounces skinless cooked chicken breast, 1 slice of Swiss cheese and 1 small sourdough roll

OPTION 3 (¼) (½)

Salad made with 2 cups Romaine lettuce, 2 ounces skinless cooked chicken breast, ½ cup chickpeas, ¼ cup apple slices, 2-3 thin slices avocado, 2 Tbsp shredded cheddar cheese and 2 Tbs salad dressing

OPTION 4 (½)

Rice bowl made with 1 cup brown rice, 3 ounces skinless cooked chicken breast, ½ cup broccoli sautéed in 1 tsp canola oil and ¼ cup black beans

OPTION 5   🍞🍞 (1¼🥦) 🥛🥛

1 slice store-bought pizza topped with 1 cup vegetables, ¼ cup tomato sauce and 2 ounces mozzarella cheese

OPTION 6   🍞🍞 🥩🥩🥩 🥚🥚 (½🥦) 🍎

Turkey sandwich made with 2 slices whole-wheat bread, 3 ounces low-sodium turkey breast, 2 tsp mayonnaise and 2-3 slices lettuce and tomato + 1 medium apple

OPTION 7   🥩🥩🥩 🥚🥚 🍞🍞 (¾🥦) 🥛

Tuna melt made with 4 ounces tuna (albacore or white), 2 tsp mayonnaise, 1 whole-wheat English muffin, toasted, 2 slices tomato and 1 slice Swiss cheese, melted + 6 baby carrots

DINNER

OPTION 1   (1½🥦) 🥩🥩🥩 (3¼🥚) 🍞

Italian-Style Tuna with Fresh Cherry Tomato Sauce (see page 221) + mixed green salad made with 2 cups mixed greens, 2 tsp olive oil and 1-2 Tbs balsamic vinegar + 1 small sourdough or whole-grain roll

OPTION 2   🥩🥩🥩 🥦 (1½🥚) 🍞

4 ounces baked salmon made with 1 tsp olive oil + 2 portions **Shredded Brussels Sprouts (see page 233)** + ½ cup brown rice

OPTION 3   🍞🍞 🥩🥩🥩 🥦 🥚🥚 (½🥛)

Shrimp pasta made with 1 cup penne pasta, 4 ounces steamed shrimp, 1 cup eggplant and tomato sautéed in 2 tsp olive oil + 2 Tbs grated Parmesan cheese

OPTION 4

Spaghetti and meatballs made with 1 cup cooked whole-wheat spaghetti, 2-3 small chicken, turkey or beef meatballs, ½ cup tomato sauce + 2 Tbs grated Parmesan cheese + baked kale chips made with 1 cup fresh kale sautéed with 1 tsp olive oil + seasonings

OPTION 5

Bean and chicken quesadilla made with 2 corn tortillas, 3 ounces skinless cooked chicken breast, ½ cup black beans, 2 Tbs shredded cheddar cheese + ¼ cup guacamole

OPTION 6

Lentil fajita made with 1 small flour tortilla, ½ cup lentils and ¼ cup shredded cheddar cheese + 1 cup broccoli sautéed with 2 tsp olive oil and garlic

OPTION 7

Chicken vegetable stir-fry made with 3 ounces skinless cooked chicken breast, 1½ cups mixed vegetables (broccoli, zucchini, yellow squash, green pepper and/or onion), 2 Tbs hoisin sauce and 2 tsp canola oil + 1 cup cooked brown rice

SNACK

OPTION 1

Blueberries with Ricotta Cream (see page 236) + ½ ounce (7 halves) walnuts

OPTION 2

1 cup nonfat Greek yogurt + ½ ounce (24 whole) pistachios

OPTION 3 (½) (50-calorie)

Chocolate Walnut Granola Bar (see page 237)

OPTION 4 (½)

Popcorn with "Fake" Cheese Topping (see page 239) + ½ ounce (12) almonds + 1 clementine

OPTION 5 (64-calorie) (½)

1 cup nonfat Greek yogurt topped with 1 Tbs honey + ½ cup sliced strawberries

OPTION 6

Cheese and crackers made with 5 Triscuits and 1 ounce (1 slice) Swiss cheese

OPTION 7

1 cup nonfat plain yogurt topped with 1 cup blueberries

GLOSSARY

VITAL NUTRIENTS

Biotin is a water-soluble B vitamin that works with several enzymes to turn carbohydrates into energy, produce fatty acids, and create or metabolize amino acids. It also supports the functions of deoxyribonucleic acid (DNA), the body's basic genetic material. And biotin promotes healthy skin, hair and nails.

Calcium is a major mineral that, with vitamin D and phosphorus, helps maintain strong bones and teeth. It also helps muscles contract and blood vessels relax and constrict. And calcium transmits nerve impulses and helps enzymes and hormones function properly.

Chloride is a major mineral that works with sodium and potassium to regulate water balance in the body. It is also a key component of gastric juices (hydrochloric acid) and salt (sodium chloride). In addition, chloride helps create nerve impulses and supports immune function.

Choline, which is neither a vitamin nor a mineral, is an essential nutrient needed to create acetylcholine, a neurotransmitter involved in muscle control and memory. It also helps maintain the structure of cell membranes and metabolize and transport fats.

Chromium is a trace mineral that helps the hormone insulin function properly to maintain normal blood glucose levels. It also helps release energy from carbohydrates and fats, and it plays a role in immune function.

Copper is a trace mineral that works as part of several enzymes to support many vital bodily functions, such as the creation of energy, the formation of connective tissue, the metabolism of iron and the production of red blood cells. In addition, it plays a role in the maintenance of the brain and nervous system function. Copper is also needed to make melanin, the pigment that colors our hair, skin and eyes.

Fluoride is a trace mineral that is essential for maintaining strong bones and teeth (especially tooth enamel) and preventing dental caries.

Folate is a water-soluble B vitamin that facilitates the production of red blood cells and DNA, the body's genetic material. It also helps the body metabolize proteins, and it helps the cells of the body grow and divide. Furthermore, folate plays a part in the creation of several brain chemicals, including serotonin, which regulate mood and sleep. It may also prevent or slow the cognitive decline that occurs with age, and it works with other B vitamins to help regulate levels of homocysteine (an amino acid), which serves to reduce the risk of heart disease and stroke, and possibly Alzheimer's disease.

Iodine is a trace mineral that is a key component of two thyroid hormones that regulate body temperature, basal metabolic rate, reproduction and growth.

Iron is a trace mineral that helps hemoglobin, a protein found in red blood cells, and myoglobin, a protein found in muscles, shuttle oxygen to various parts of the body. It is also part of many enzymes (proteins that speed chemical reactions and create energy), and it plays a role in the synthesis of collagen, amino acids, neurotransmitters and hormones.

Magnesium is major mineral that helps muscles contract and relax, supports bone health, helps regulate body temperature and helps build protein.

Manganese is an essential trace mineral that is part of, or works with, several enzymes to create fatty acids and cholesterol, as well as bones, collagen and connective tissue. It is also part of a key enzyme that protects the body against damage caused by free radicals.

Molybdenum is a trace mineral needed by many enzymes in the body to help them function properly. It supports a healthy nervous system, creates energy in cells and processes wastes in the kidneys.

Niacin, also known as vitamin B_3, is a water-soluble vitamin that helps the body create energy from carbohydrates and fatty acids. It works with many enzymes (proteins) in several important chemical reactions. It also supports healthy skin, digestion and nerve function.

Pantothenic Acid, a water-soluble B vitamin, creates energy from carbohydrates, fat and protein. It also aids in the production of hormones, essential fats and cholesterol.

Phosphorus is a major mineral that helps all cells of the body function optimally. It works with calcium and vitamin D to build and maintain strong bones and teeth. It also helps create energy from food, maintain acid/base balance and deliver oxygen to various body tissues. In addition, phosphorus is a key component of DNA, ribonucleic acid (RNA) and phospholipids, which have important functions in the body.

Potassium, a major mineral found in every cell of the body, helps regulate fluid balance (along with sodium and chloride), helps transport nerve signals and helps muscles—including the heart—contract.

Riboflavin, also known as vitamin B_2, is a water-soluble vitamin that plays a role in turning carbohydrates into energy. It aids in the production of red blood cells, which carry oxygen around the body, and is involved in several important chemical reactions in the body. It also helps convert tryptophan into niacin, supports healthy skin and helps maintain vision.

Selenium is an important antioxidant mineral that fights damage to cells caused by free radicals. It also helps maintain thyroid function and supports immune function.

Sodium is a major mineral that works with potassium, chloride and other minerals to maintain fluid balance in the body. It also helps regulate blood pressure; helps muscles, including the heart muscle, contract and relax; and transmits nerve impulses.

Sulfur is a mineral that supports healthy joints, skin, hair, nails and connective tissues. Sulfur may also play a role in reducing pain by slowing nerve impulses.

Thiamine, also known as vitamin B_1, is a water-soluble vitamin that helps the body use carbohydrates for energy. It also helps enzymes maintain the functions of the muscles, nerves and the heart. Thiamine is needed, too, for healthy skin and nails.

Vitamin A is a fat-soluble vitamin that helps create and maintain healthy teeth, bones and soft body tissues. It supports healthy skin and vision, and it strengthens the immune system.

Vitamin B_6, also known as pyroxidine, is a water-soluble vitamin that works with many enzymes that perform several chemical reactions in the body. It breaks down glycogen (stored glucose) and helps form heme, the iron-containing part of hemoglobin, which is found in red blood cells, through which oxygen is delivered around the body. It also contributes to the production of neurotransmitters.

Vitamin B_{12} is a water-soluble vitamin that helps the body produce energy from food. In addition, it assists in the formation of red blood cells and deoxyribonucleic acid (DNA), the body's basic genetic material. It also supports a healthy nervous system by working with enzymes and other B vitamins to create serotonin and other neurotransmitters. And vitamin B_{12} also helps metabolize folate.

Vitamin C is a water-soluble vitamin that works as an antioxidant, protecting cells of the body against free radical damage. It also helps create collagen, the body's main structural protein, which holds skin, bones and other tissues together, supports healthy gums and helps wounds heal. Vitamin C supports a healthy immune system as well, and helps the body absorb iron from food. And it plays a role in the creation of norepinephrine, a brain chemical that affects mood.

Vitamin D is a fat-soluble vitamin that helps control the level of calcium and phosphorus in the blood and thus is instrumental in building and maintaining strong bones and teeth.

Vitamin E is a fat-soluble vitamin that plays an important role as an antioxidant. It protects vitamins A and C, red blood cells and essential fatty acids from being destroyed by free radicals. It also helps form red blood cells and facilitates the body's use of vitamin K.

Vitamin K is a fat-soluble vitamin needed by the liver to help it create several proteins required for blood to clot. It also supports proteins involved in bone metabolism and cell growth.

Zinc is a trace mineral that plays a key role in growth and sexual development, and it also helps proteins (such as enzymes and hormones) function. In addition, it aids in the production of deoxyribonucleic acid (DNA), the body's genetic material. Zinc also helps the body maintain smell and taste, and it supports a healthy immune system.

APPENDIX A

ACTIVITY CONVERSION CHART FOR WOMEN

Here's a guide to help you count the steps taken while doing some of your favorite activities.

Activity	Steps Per 10 Minutes	Activity	Steps Per 10 Minutes
Aerobic dancing, low impact	1790	Bicycling, stationary, 200 watts, vigorous effort	3760
Aerobics, high impact	2510	Bowling	1070
Aerobics, 6-8" step	3040	Canoeing	1430
Aerobics, 10-12" step	3580	Chopping wood	2150
Aerobics, water	1430	Circuit training, general	2860
Backpacking, 0-9 lb. load	2510	Dancing, slow ballroom	1070
Backpacking, 10-20 lb. load	2690	Dancing, fast ballroom	1610
Ballet or modern, twist, jazz, tap, jitterbug	1720	Elliptical, general	2860
Baseball or softball, fast or slow pitch, general	1790	Football, competitive	3220
Basketball, nongame	2150	Football, touch or flag	2860
Basketball, game	2860	Gardening, moderate	1610
Basketball, wheelchair	2330	Gardening, heavy	1790
Bicycling, BMX or mountain	3040	Golfing, without cart	1610
Bicycling, general	2860	Golfing, riding in cart	1250
Bicycling, stationary, 100 watts, light effort	1970	Hiking	2150
Bicycling, stationary, 150 watts, moderate effort	2510	Horseshoes	1070

Activity	Steps Per 10 Minutes	Activity	Steps Per 10 Minutes
Ice-skating	2510	Snowboarding	2330
Jogging, general	2510	Snowshoeing	2860
Jogging, water	2860	Soccer, casual	2510
Judo, jujitsu, karate, kickboxing, tae kwon do	3580	Soccer, competitive	3580
Jumping rope, slow	2860	Stair climber machine	3220
Jumping rope, moderate	3580	Stair climbing, downstairs	1070
Jumping rope, fast	4300	Stair climbing, upstairs	2860
Mowing lawn, push mower	1970	Swimming, backstroke	2510
Pilates	1250	Swimming, breaststroke	3580
Racquetball, casual	2510	Swimming, butterfly	3940
Racquetball, competitive	3580	Swimming laps, freestyle, moderate, light effort	2510
Roller-skating	2510	Swimming, sidestroke	2860
Rollerblading	4300	Tennis, singles	2860
Rowing, moderate	2510	Tennis, doubles	2150
Running, 8 mph (7.5 min/mile)	4830	Vacuuming	1250
Running, 10 mph (6 min/mile)	5730	Volleyball	1430
Scrubbing floors	1360	Walking for pleasure	1250
Shoveling snow	2150	Washing and waxing the car	1610
Skateboarding	1790	Waterskiing	2150
Skiing, cross-country	2860	Weight lifting, light or moderate	1070
Skiing, moderate downhill	2150	Wrestling	2150
		Yoga	900

Source: "Activity Conversion for Adults," America on the Move, accessed February 19, 2013, https://aom3.americaonthemove.org.

APPENDIX B

DAILY RECOMMENDED NUTRIENT INTAKES FOR WOMEN AGED 19 TO 70+

	Dietary Reference Intakes	Tolerable Upper Intake Levels (UL)[1]
Vitamins		
Vitamin A (mcg)	700	3000
Vitamin C (mg)	75	2000
Vitamin D (mcg)	15 (20 for ages 70+)	100
Vitamin E (mg)	15	1000
Vitamin K* (mcg)	90	ND[2]
Thiamine (mg)	1.1	ND[2]
Riboflavin (mg)	1.1	ND[2]
Niacin (mg)	14	35
Vitamin B_6 (mg)	1.3 (1.5 for ages 51+)	100
Folate (mcg)	400	1000
Vitamin B_{12} (mcg)	2.4	ND[2]
Pantothenic Acid* (mg)	5	ND[2]
Biotin* (mcg)	30	ND[2]
Choline* (mg)	425	3500

	Dietary Reference Intakes	Tolerable Upper Intake Levels (UL)[1]
Minerals		
Calcium (mg)	1000 (1200 for ages 51+)	2500 (2000 for ages 51+)
Chromium* (mcg)	25 (20 for ages 51+)	ND[2]
Copper (mcg)	900	10,000
Fluoride* (mg)	3	10
Iodine (mcg)	150	1100
Iron (mg)	18 (8 for ages 51+)	45
Magnesium (mg)	320 (310 for ages 19–30)	350
Manganese* (mg)	1.8	11
Molybdenum (mcg)	45	2000
Phosphorus (mg)	700	4000
Selenium (mcg)	55	400
Zinc (mg)	8	40
Potassium* (g)	4.7	ND[2]
Sodium* (mg)	2300 (1300 for ages 51-70; 1200 for ages 70+)	2300
Chloride* (g)	2.3 (2 for ages 51-70; 1.8 for ages 70+)	3.6

1 The highest level of daily nutrient intake that is likely to pose no risk of adverse health effects to almost all individuals in the general population.

2 Not determined.

*Adequate Intakes (AI); No RDA has been established, but the amount established is somewhat less firmly believed to be adequate for individuals in a group.

Source: "Dietary Reference Intake for Vitamins, Minerals, Macronutrients and Water," The National Academies Press, accessed on February 20, 2013, www.nap.edu.

APPENDIX C

DIETARY REFERENCE INTAKE (DRI) ACCEPTABLE MACRONUTRIENT DISTRIBUTION RANGES

Macronutrient	Recommendations
Carbohydrate	45-65% of energy*
Fat -n-6 polyunsaturated fatty acids (linoleic) -n-3 polyunsaturated fatty acids (linolenic) -saturated fatty acids -trans-fatty acids	20-35% of energy -5-10% of energy -0.6-1.2% of energy -As low as possible while consuming a nutritionally adequate diet -As low as possible while consuming a nutritionally adequate diet
Dietary cholesterol	As low as possible while consuming a nutritionally adequate diet
Protein	10-35% of energy

*Energy means represent calories.

Source: "Dietary Reference Intake Acceptable Macronutrient Distribution Ranges," The National Academies Press, accessed on February 20, 2013, www.nap.edu.

APPENDIX D

VITALITY DIET TEMPLATE

If you don't want to follow a set menu, or if you just want ultimate flexibility when you choose foods and beverages, here's a sample one-day template that outlines the Vitality Diet recommendations for weight loss* discussed in Chapter 12. Use the Vital Foods List on pages 192 to choose items for breakfast, lunch, dinner and a snack daily in recommended portions.

Breakfast:

- 2 Starchy Carbs
- 1 Fruit
- 1 Dairy

Lunch:

- 2 Proteins
- 1 Beans + Peas
- 1 Non-Starchy Vegetable
- 1 Healthy Fat
- 50-Calorie Treat

Snack:

- 1 Dairy
- 2 Proteins
- 2 Healthy Fats
- ½ Fruit

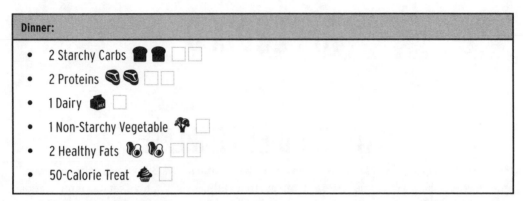

Dinner:

- 2 Starchy Carbs ☐☐
- 2 Proteins ☐☐
- 1 Dairy ☐
- 1 Non-Starchy Vegetable ☐
- 2 Healthy Fats ☐☐
- 50-Calorie Treat ☐

* If your goal is weight maintenance (rather than weight loss), consider adding at least 1 Starchy Carb, 1 Healthy Fat, $^1/_2$ Fruit and 2 Proteins or Beans and Peas daily, spread evenly throughout the day. To determine your individual calorie needs for weight loss or maintenance, find a registered dietitian nutritionist by visiting www.eatright.org.

REFERENCES

CHAPTER 1

Epel, Elissa S., Elizabeth H. Blackburn, Jue Lin, et al. 2004. "Accelerated Telomere Shortening in Response to Life Stress." *Proceedings of the National Academy of Sciences* 101(49):17312–5.

Sher, L. 2005. "Type D Personality: The Heart, Stress, and Cortisol." *QJM: An International Journal of Medicine* 98(5):323–9(7).

CHAPTER 2

Baron, Kelly G., Kathryn J. Reid, Andrew S. Kern and Phyllis C. Zee. 2011. "Role of Sleep Timing in Caloric Intake and BMI." *Obesity* 19(7):1374–8.

Carlson, Olga, Bronwen Martin, Kim S. Stote, et al. 2007. "Impact of Reduced Meal Frequency Without Caloric Restriction on Glucose Regulation in Healthy, Normal-Weight Middle-Aged Men and Women." *Metabolism* 56(12):1729–34.

Childs, Emma, Sean O'Connor and Harriet De Witt. 2011. "Bidirectional Interactions Between Acute Psychosocial Stress and Acute Intravenous Alcohol in Healthy Men." *Alcoholism: Clinical and Experimental Research* 35(10):1794–1803.

Crispim, Cibele Apareecida, Iona Zalcman Zimberg, Bruno Gomes dos Reis, Rafael Marques Diniz, Sergio Tufik and Marco Tulio de Mello. 2011. "Relationship Between Food Intake and Sleep Pattern in Healthy Individuals." *Journal of Clinical Sleep Medicine* 7(6):659–64.

Guyuron, Bahman, David J. Rowe, Adam Bryce Weinfeld, et al. 2009. "Factors Contributing to the Facial Aging of Identical Twins." *Plastic and Reconstructive Surgery* 123(4):1321–31.

Noordam, Raymond, David A. Gunn, Cyrena C. Tomlin, et al. 2013. "High Serum Glucose Levels Are Associated With a Higher Perceived Age." *AGE* 35(1):189–95.

Sharma, Satyasheel, Maria Fernanda Fernandes and Stephanie Fulton. 2012. "Adaptations in Brain Reward Circuitry Underlie Palatable Food Cravings and Anxiety Induced by High-Fat Diet Withdrawal." *International Journal of Obesity* doi: 10.1038/ijo.2012.197.

CHAPTER 3

The American Cancer Society. "Acrylamide." Accessed March 31, 2013. www.cancer.org/cancer/cancercauses/othercarcinogens/athome/acrylamide

Albertson, Ann M., A. Christine Wold and Nandan Joshi. 2012. "Ready-to-Eat Cereal Consumption Patterns: The Relationship to Nutrient Intake, Whole Grain Intake, and Body Mass Index in an Older American Population." *Journal of Aging Research* 2012:631310.

Barr, Susan I., Loretta Difrancesco, Victor L. Fulgoni III. 2013."Consumption of Breakfast and the Type of Breakfast Consumed Are Positively Associated with Nutrient Intakes and Adequacy of Canadian Adults." *The Journal of Nutrition* 143(1):86–92.

Batres-Marquez, S. Patricia, Helen H. Jensen and Julie Upton. 2009. "Rice Consumption in the United States: Recent Evidence from Food Consumption Surveys." *Journal of the American Dietetic Association* 109(10):1719–27.

Berti, Christiana, Patrizia Riso, Antonella Brusamolino and Marisa Porrini. 2005. "Effect on Appetite Control of Minor Cereal and Pseudocereal Products." *British Journal of Nutrition* 94(5):850–8.

Christopher, J. and Caroline S. Fox. 2010. "Whole- and Refined-Grain Intakes are Differentially Associated with Abdominal Visceral and Subcutaneous Adiposity in Healthy Adults: The Framingham Heart Study." *The American Journal of Clinical Nutrition* 92(5):1165–71.

Colditz, Graham. 2003. "Relation Between Changes in Intakes of Dietary Fiber and Grain Products and Changes in Weight and Development of Obesity Among Middle-Aged Women." *American Journal of Clinical Nutrition* 78(5):920–27.

Consumer Reports Magazine. 2012. "Arsenic In Your Food." *Consumer Reports Magazine.* Accessed February 1, 2013. www.consumerreports.org/cro/magazine/2012/11/arsenic-in-your-food/index.htm

Cosgrove, Maeve, Oscar Franco, Stewart Granger, Peter Murray and Andrew Mayes. 2007. "Dietary Nutrient Intakes and Skin-Aging Appearance Among Middle-Aged American Women." *American Journal of Clinical Nutrition* 86(4):1225–31.

Deshmukh-Taskar, Priya, Theresa A. Nicklas, John D. Radcliffe, Carole E. O'Neil and Yan Liu. 2012. "The Relationship of Breakfast Skipping and Type of Breakfast Consumed With Overweight/Obesity, Abdominal Obesity, Other Cardiometabolic Risk Factors and the Metabolic Syndrome in Young Adults. The National Health and Nutrition Examination Survey (NHANES): 1999-2006." *Public Health Nutrition* Oct:1–10.

Flugoni III, Victor, Julie L. Upton, Sally A. Fulgoni and Maggie Moon. 2010. "Diet Quality and Markers for Human Health in Rice Eaters Versus Non–Rice Eaters." *Nutrition Today* 45(6):262–72.

Gaesser, Glen A. 2007. "Carbohydrate Quantity and Quality in Relation to Body Mass Index." *Journal of the American Dietetic Association* 107(10):1768–80.

Good, Carolyn K., Norton Holschuh, Ann M. Albertson and Allison L. Eldridge. 2008. "Whole Grain Consumption and Body Mass Index in Adult Women: An Analysis of NHANES 1999-2000 and the USDA Pyramid Servings Database." *Journal of the American College of Nutrition* (27)1:80–7.

Grandjean, Ann, Victor L. Fulgoni III, Kristin J. Reimers and Sanjiv Agarwal. 2008. "Popcorn Consumption and Dietary and Physiological Parameters of US Children and Adults: Analysis of the National Health and Nutrition Examination Survey (NHANES) 1999-2002 Dietary Survey Data." *Journal of the American Dietetic Association* 108(5):853–6.

Grotto, David. 2013. *The Best Things You Can Eat: For Everything from Aches to Zzzz, the Definitive Guide to the Nutrition-Packed Foods that Energize, Heal, and Help You Look Great.* Cambridge, MA:Da Capo Lifelong Books.

Hu, Emily A., An Pan, Vasanti Malik and Qi Sun. 2012. "White Rice Consumption and Risk of Type 2 Diabetes: Meta-Analysis and Systematic Review." *British Medical Journal* 344:e1454.

Institute of Medicine. 2002-2005. *Dietary Reference Intakes for Energy, Carbohydrate, Fiber, Fat, Fatty Acids, Cholesterol, Protein, and Amino Acids.* www.nap.edu.

Irby, Susan. 2012. *Complete Idiot's Guide to Quinoa.* New York: ALPHA.

Kemppainen, Tarja A., Markku T. Heikkinen, Matti K. Ristikankare, Veli-Matti Kosma and Risto Julkunen. 2010. "Nutrient Intakes During Diets Including Unkilned and Large Amounts of Oats in Celiac Disease." *European Journal of Clinical Nutrition* 64(1): 62–7.

Lee, Ann R., D.L. Ng, E. Dave, E.J. Ciaccio and P.H. Green. 2009. "The Effect of Substituting Alternative Grains in the Diet on the Nutritional Profile of the Gluten-Free Diet." *Journal of Human Nutrition and Dietetics* 22(4):359–63.

Merchant, Anwar T., Hassanali Vatanparast, Shahzaib Barlas, et al. 2009. "Carbohydrate Intake and Overweight and Obesity Among Healthy Adults." *Journal of the American Dietetic Association* 109(7):1165–72.

Mozaffarian, Dariush, Tao Hao, Eric B. Rimm, Walter C. Willett and Frank B. Hu. 2011. "Changes in Diet and Lifestyle and Long-Term Weight Gain in Women and Men." *New England Journal of Medicine* 364(25):2392–404.

Newgent, Jackie. 2012. *1000 Low-Calorie Recipes.* Hoboken: Wiley.

Nguyen, Von, Lisa Cooper, Joshua Lowndes, et al. 2012. "Popcorn is More Satiating Than Potato Chips in Normal-Weight Adults." *Nutrition Journal* 11:71.

Qing Ye, Eva, Sara A. Chacko, Elizabeth L. Chou, Matthew Kugizaki and Simin Liu. 2012. "Greater Whole-Grain Intake is Associated with Lower Risk of Type 2 Diabetes, Cardiovascular Disease, and Weight Gain." *Journal of Nutrition* 142(7):1304–13.

Slavin, Joanne L. 2005. "Dietary Fiber and Body Weight." *Nutrition* 21(3):411–8.

Soriguer, Federico, Natalia Colomo, Gabriel Olveira, et al. 2012. "White Rice Consumption and Risk of Type 2 Diabetes." *Clinical Nutrition* doi:10.1016/j.clnu.2012.11.008.

Turski, Michal P., Piotr Kaminski, Wojciech Zgrajka, Monika Turska and Waldemar A. Turski. 2012. "Potato–An Important Source of Nutritional Kynurenic Acid." *Plant Foods for Human Nutrition* 67(1):17–23.

U.S. Department of Agriculture, Agricultural Research Service. 2012. "Energy Intakes: Percentages of Energy from Protein, Carbohydrate, Fat, and Alcohol, by Gender and Age, What We Eat in America, NHANES 2009-2010." Accessed February 10, 2013. www.ars.usda.gov/ba/bhnrc/fsrg

Vega-Gálvez, Antonio, Margarita Miranda, Judith Vergara, Elsa Uribe, Luis Puente and Enrique A. Martínez. 2010. "Nutrition Facts and Functional Potential of Quinoa (Chenopodium quinoa willd.), an Ancient Andean Grain: a Review." *Journal of the Science of Food and Agriculture* 90(15):2541–7.

Visoli, Francesco, Catalina Alarcon De La Lastra and Cristina Andres-Lacueva, et al. 2011. "Polyphenols and Human Health: a Prospectus." *Critical Reviews in Food Science* 51(6):524–46.

Waller, Sandia, Jillon Vander Wal, David Klurfeld, et al. 2004. "Evening Ready-to-Eat Cereal Consumption Contributes to Weight Management." *Journal of the American College of Nutrition* 23(4):316–21.

Williams, Peter G. 2012. "Evaluation of the Evidence Between Consumption of Refined Grains and Health Outcomes." *Nutrition Review* 70(2):80–99.

Wurtman, Judith, and Frusztajer Marquis. 2006. *The Serotonin Power Diet: Use Your Brain's Natural Chemistry to Cut Cravings, Curb Emotional Overeating, and Lose Weight.* Emmau, PA: Rodale.

Young, Lisa. 2006. *The Portion Teller Plan.* New York: Three Rivers Press.

CHAPTER 4

American Heart Association. "Healthy Diet Goals." Accessed October 10, 2012. www.heart.org/HEARTORG/GettingHealthy/NutritionCenter/HealthyDietGoals/Healthy-Diet-Goals_UCM_310436_SubHomePage.jsp

Bes-Rastrollo, Maira, Nicole M. Wedick, Miguel Angel Martinez-Gonzalez, Tricia Y. Li, Laura Sampson and Frank B. Hu. 2009. "Prospective Study of Nut Consumption, Long-Term Weight Change, and Obesity Risk in Women." *The American Journal of Clinical Nutrition* 89(6):1913–9.

Bolling, Bradley W., Oliver Chen, Diane McKay and Jeffrey B. Blumberg. 2011. "Tree Nut Phytochemicals: Composition, Antioxidant Capacity, Bioactivity, Impact Factors. A Systematic Review of Almonds, Brazils, Cashews, Hazelnuts, Macadamias, Pecans, Pine Nuts, Pistachios and Walnuts." *Nutrition Research Reviews* 24(2):244–75.

Bowman, G.L., L.C. Silbert, D. Howieson, et al. 2011. "Nutrient Biomarker Patterns, Cognitive Function, and MRI Measures of Brain Aging." *Neurology* 78(4):241–9.

Carlsen, Monica H., Bente L. Halvorsen, Kari Holte, et al. 2010. "The Total Antioxidant Content of More Than 3100 Foods, Beverages, Spices, Herbs and Supplements Used Worldwide." *Nutrition Journal* 9(3) doi:10.1186/1475–2891–9–3.

Fernández-Montero, Alejandro, Maira Bes-Rastrollo, Juan J. Beunza, et al. 2012. "Nut Consumption and Incidence of Metabolic Syndrome After 6-year Follow-up: the SUN (Seguimiento Universidad de Navarra, University of Navarra Follow-up) Cohort." *Public Health Nutrition* 23:1–9.

Foxcroft, David, L. Ryan and C. Sanhueza. 2013. "Diet and the Risk of Unipolar Depression in Adults: Systematic Review of Cohort Studies." *Journal of Human Nutrition and* Dietetics 26(1):56–70.

Franco, Oscar, Frank B. Hu, Francesca Crowe, et al. 2012. "Association Between Fish Consumption, Long Chain Omega 3 Fatty Acids, and Risk of Cerebrovascular Disease: Systematic Review and Meta-Analysis." *British Medical Journal* 345: e6698.

Griel, Amy E. and Penny M. Kris-Etherton. 2006. "Tree Nuts and the Lipid Profile: a Review of Clinical Studies." *British Journal of Nutrition* (96) 2:S68–78.

Heller, Samantha. 2010. *Get Smart: Samantha Heller's Nutrition Prescription for Boosting Brain Power and Optimizing Total Body Health*. Baltimore: The Johns Hopkins University Press.

Helm, Janet. 2012. *Cooking Light The Food Lover's Healthy Habits Cookbook: Great Food & Expert Advice That Will Change Your Life*. Alabama: Oxmoor House.

Hughes, Maria Celia B., Gail M. Williams, Anny Fourtanier and Adele C. Green. 2009. "Food Intake, Dietary Patterns, and Actinic Keratoses of the Skin: a Longitudinal Study." *The American Journal of Clinical Nutrition* 89(4):1246–55.

Institute of Medicine. 2002–2005. *Dietary Reference Intakes for Energy, Carbohydrate, Fiber, Fat, Fatty Acids, Cholesterol, Protein, and Amino Acids*. www.nap.edu.

Kelly Jr., John H. and Joan Sabate. 2006. "Nuts and Coronary Heart Disease: an Epidemiological Perspective." *British Journal of Nutrition* (96)2:S61–7.

Kiecolt-Glaser, Janice K., Martha A. Belury, Kyle Porter, David Q. Beversdorf, Stanley Lemeshow and Ronald Glaser. 2007. "Depressive Symptoms, Omega-6:Omega-3 Fatty Acids, and Inflammation in Older Adults." *Psychosomatic Medicine* 69(3):217–24.

Kromhout, Daan. 2012. "Omega-3 Fatty Acids and Coronary Heart Disease. The Final Verdict?" *Current Opinion in Lipidology* 23(6):554–9.

Lucas, Michael, Fariba Marzaei, Eilis J. O'Reilly, et al. 2011. "Dietary Intake of n–3 and n–6 Fatty Acids and the Risk of Clinical Depression in Women: a 10-y Prospective Follow-Up Study." *The American Journal of Clinical Nutrition* 93(6):1337–43.

Mattes, Richard D. and Mark L. Dreher. 2010. "Nuts and Healthy Body Weight Maintenance Mechanisms." *Asia Pacific Journal of Clinical Nutrition* 19(1):137–41.

Mukuddem-Petersen, Welma Oosthuizen and Johann C. Jerling. 2005. "A Systematic Review of the Effects of Nuts on Blood Lipid Profiles in Humans." *The Journal of Nutrition* 135(9):2082–9.

Nicholson, Tiffany, Haidar Khademi and Mohammed H. Moghadasian. 2013. "The Role of Marine n–3 Fatty Acids in Improving Cardiovascular Health: A Review." *Food & Function* 4(3):357–65.

O'Neil, Carole E., Debra R. Keast, Theresa A. Nicklas and Victor L. Fulgoni. 2012. "Out-of-hand Nut Consumption is Associated with Improved Nutrient Intake and Health Risk Markers in U.S. Children and Adults: National Health and Nutrition Examination Survey 1999–2004." *Nutrition Research* 32(3):185–94.

O'Neil, Carole E., Debra R. Keast, Theresa A. Nicklas and Victor L. Fulgoni. 2011. "Nut Consumption is Associated with Decreased Health Risk Factors for Cardiovascular Disease and Metabolic Syndrome in U.S. Adults: NHANES 1999-2004." *Journal of the American College of Nutrition* 30(6):502–10.

O'Neil, Carole E., Debra R. Keast, Theresa A. Nicklas and Victor L. Fulgoni. 2010. "Tree Nut Consumption Improves Nutrient Intake and Diet Quality in U.S. Adults: An Analysis of National Health and Nutrition Examination Survey (NHANES) 1999–2004." *Asia Pacific Journal of Clinical Nutrition* 19(1):142–50.

Ros, Emilio, Linda C. Tapsell and Joan Sabate. 2010. "Nuts and Berries for Heart Health." *Current Atherosclerosis Reports* 12(6):397–406.

Simopoulos, Artemis P. 2008. "The Importance of the Omega-6/Omega-3 Fatty Acid Ratio in Cardiovascular Disease and Other Chronic Diseases." *Experimental Biology and Medicine* 223(6):674–8.

U.S. Department of Agriculture and U.S. Department of Health and Human Services. 2010. *Dietary Guidelines for Americans, 2010*. 7th Edition, Washington, DC: U.S. Government Printing Office, December 2010.

CHAPTER 5

Abeysekara, Saman, Phillip D. Chilibeck, Hassanali Vatanparast and Gordon A. Zello. 2012. "A Pulse-Based Diet is Effective for Reducing Total and LDL-Cholesterol in Older Adults." *British Journal of Nutrition* 108 (Suppl 1):S103–10.

American Heart Association and National Cholesterol Education Program. "Healthy Diet Goals." www.heart.org/HEARTORG/GettingHealthy/NutritionCenter/HealthyDietGoals/Healthy-Diet-Goals_UCM_310436_SubHomePage.jsp

Asp, M.L., J.R. Richardson, A.L. Collene, K.R. Droll and M.A. Belury. 2012. "Dietary Protein and Beef Consumption Predict for Markers of Muscle Mass and Nutrition Status in Older Adults." *Journal of Nutrition, Health, and Aging* 16(9):784–90.

Bazzano, Lydia A., Angela M. Thompson, Michael T. Tees, Cuong H. Nguyen and Donna M. Winham. 2012. "Non-Soy Legume Consumption Lowers Cholesterol Levels: A Meta-Analysis of Randomized Controlled Trials." *Nutrition, Metabolism, and Cardiovascular Diseases* 21(2):94–103.

Castelo-Branco, C. and M.J. Cancelo Hidalgo. 2011. "Isoflavones: Effects On Bone Health." *Clinacteric* 14(2):204–11.

Chen, X., Y. Huang and H.G. Cheng. 2012. "Lower Intake of Vegetables and Legumes Associated with Cognitive Decline Among Illiterate Elderly Chinese: A 3-year Cohort Study." *Journal of Nutrition, Health, and Aging* 16(6):549–52.

Cope, M.B., J.W. Erdman Jr. and D.B. Allison. 2008. "The Potential Role of Soyfoods in Weight and Adiposity Reduction: An Evidence-Based Review." *Obesity Review* 9(3):219–35.

Darmadi-Blackberry, Irene, Mark L. Wahlqvist, Antigone Kouris-Blazos, et al. 2004. "Legumes: The Most Important Dietary Predictor of Survival in Older People of Different Ethnicities." *Asia Pacific Journal of Clinical Nutrition* 13(2):217–20.

Fallaize, Rosalind, Louise Wilson, Juliet Gray, Linda M. Morgan and Bruce A. Griffin. 2012. "Variation in the Effects of Three Different Breakfast Meals on Subjective Satiety and Subsequent Intake of Energy at Lunch and Evening Meal." *European Journal of Nutrition* 52(4):1353–9.

He, Ka, Anwar Merchant, Eric B. Rimm, et al. 2003. "Dietary Fat Intake and Risk of Stroke in Male US Healthcare Professionals: 14 Year Prospective Cohort Study." *British Medical Journal* 327(7418): 777–82.

Hutchins, Andrea, Donna Winham and Sharon Thompson. 2012. "Phaseolus Beans: Impact on Glycaemic Response and Chronic Disease Risk in Human Subjects." *British Journal of Nutrition* S1:S52–S65.

Institute of Medicine. 2002–2005. *Dietary Reference Intakes for Energy, Carbohydrate, Fiber, Fat, Fatty Acids, Cholesterol, Protein, and Amino Acids*. www.nap.edu.

Kim, Sun-Young, Su-Jong Kim, Jin-Young Lee, et al. 2004. "Protective Effects of Dietary Soy Isoflavones Against UV-Induced Skin-Aging in Hairless Mouse Model." *Journal of American College of Nutrition* 23(2):157–62.

Lanou, Amy J. 2011. "Soy Foods: Are They Useful for Optimal Bone Health?" *Thereaputic Advances in Musculoskeletal Disease* 3(6):293–300.

Li, Yanfeng, Qi Dai, Stuart H. Tedders, Cassandra Arroyo and Jian Zhang. 2010. "Legume Consumption and Severe Depressed Mood, the Modifying Roles of Gender and Menopausal Status." *Public Health Nutrition* 13(8):1198–1206.

Micha, Renata, Sarah Wallace and Dariush Mozaffarian. 2010. "Red and Processed Meat Consumption and Risk of Incident Coronary Heart Disease, Stroke, and Diabetes: A Systematic Review and Meta-Analysis." *Circulation* 121(21):2271–83.

Michelfelder, Aaron J. 2009. "Soy: A Complete Source of Protein." *American Family Physician* 79(1):43–7.

Mitchell, Diane C., Frank R. Lawrence, Terryl J. Hartman and Julianne M. Curran. 2009. "Consumption of Dry Beans, Peas, and Lentils Could Improve Diet Quality in the US Population." *Journal of the American Dietetic Association* 109(5):909–13.

Morris, Martha S. and Paul F. Jacques. 2012. "Total Protein, Animal Protein and Physical Activity in Relation to Muscle Mass in Middle-Aged and Older Americans." *British Journal of Nutrition* 109(7):1294–303.

National Institutes of Health. 2002. *Third Report of the National Cholesterol Education Program (NCEP) Expert Panel on Detection, Evaluation, and Treatment of High Blood Cholesterol in Adults (Adult Treatment Panel III)*. 02–5215.

Nicklas, Theresa A., Carole E. O'Neil, Michael Zanovec, Debra Keast and Victor L. Fulgoni III. 2012. "Contribution of Beef Consumption to Nutrient Intake, Diet Quality, and Food Patterns in the Diets of the US Population." *Meat Science* 90(1):152–8.

Papanikolaou, Yanni and Victor L. Fulgoni III. 2008. "Bean Consumption is Associated With Greater Nutrient Intake, Reduced Systolic Blood Pressure, Lower Body Weight, and a Smaller Waist Circumference in Adults: Results From the National Health and Nutrition Examination Survey 1999–2002." *Journal of the American College of Nutrition* 27(5):569–76.

Pombo-Rodrigues S., W. Calame and R. Re. 2011. "The Effects of Consuming Eggs for Lunch on Satiety and Subsequent Food Intake." *International Journal of Food Sciences and Nutrition* 62(6):593–9.

Ratliff, Joseph, Jose O. Leite, Ryan de Ogburn, et al. 2010. "Consuming Eggs for Breakfast Influences Plasma Glucose and Ghrelin, While Reducing Energy Intake During the Next 24 Hours in Adult Men." *Nutrition Research* 30(2):96–103.

Roussell, Michael A., Alison M. Hill and Trent L. Gaugler. 2012. "Beef in an Optimal Lean Diet Study: Effects on Lipids, Lipoproteins, and Apolipoproteins." *American Journal of Clinical Nutrition* 95(1):9–16.

Santesso, N., E.A. Akl, M. Bianchi, A. Mente, R. Mustafa, D. Heels-Ansdell and H.J. Schünemann. 2012. "Effects of Higher-Versus Lower-Protein Diets on Health Outcomes: A Systematic Review and Meta-Analysis." *European Journal of Clinical Nutrition* 66(7):780–8.

Sievenpiper, J.L., C.W.C. Kendall, A. Esfahani, et al. 2009. "Effect of Non-Oil-Seed Pulses on Glycaemic Control: a Systematic Review and Meta-Analysis of Randomised Controlled Experimental Trials in People With and Without Diabetes." *Diabetologia* 52(8):1479–95.

Symons, T. Brock, Scott E. Schutzler, Tara L. Cocke, Robert R. Wolfe and Douglas Paddon-Jones. 2007. "Aging Does Not Impair the Anabolic Response to a Protein-Rich Meal." *American Journal of Clinical Nutrition* 86(2):451–6.

Symons, T. Brock, Melinda Sheffield-Moore, Robert R. Wolfe and Douglas Paddon-Jones. 2009. "A Moderate Serving of High-Quality Protein Maximally Stimulates Skeletal Muscle Protein Synthesis in Young and Elderly Subjects." *Journal of the American Dietetic Association* 109(9):1582–6.

CHAPTER 6

Bowman, Gene L., Lisa C. Silbert, Hiroko Dodge, et al. 2012. "Nutrient Biomarker Patterns, Cognitive Function, and MRI Measures of Brain Aging." *Neurology* 78(4):241–9.

Chocano-Bedoya, Patricia O., JoAnne E. Manson, Susan E. Hackinson, et al. 2011. "Dietary B Vitamin Intake and Incident Premenstrual Syndrome." *American Journal of Clinical Nutrition* 93(5):1080–6.

Hvas, Anne-Mette, Svend Juul, Per Bech and Ebba Nexo. 2004. "Vitamin B_6 Level is Associated with Symptoms of Depression." *Psychotherapy and Psychosomatics* 73(6):340–3.

Hwang, Ji-Yun, Sang Eun Lee, Sun Hye Kim, Hye Won Chung and Wha Young Kim. 2010. "Psychological Distress is Associated with Inadequate Dietary Intake in Vietnamese Marriage Immigrant Women in Korea." *Journal of the American Dietetic Association* 110(5):779–85.

Mishra, Gita D., Sarah A. McNaughton, Maria A. O'Connell, Celia J. Pyrnna and Diana Kuh. 2009. "Intake of B Vitamins in Childhood and Adult Life in Relation to Psychological Distress Among Women in a British Birth Cohort." *Public Health Nutrition* 12(2):166–74.

Skarupski, Kimberly A., Christine Tangney, Hong Li, Bichun Ouyang, Denis A. Evans and Martha Clare Morris. 2010. "Longitudinal Association of Vitamin B-6, Folate, and Vitamin B-12 with Depressive Symptoms Among Older Adults Over Time." *American Journal of Clinical Nutrition* 92(2):330–35.

Tangney, Christy C., N.T. Aggarwal, H. Li, et al. 2011. "Vitamin B_{12}, Cognition, and Brain MRI Measures: A Cross-Sectional Examination." *Neurology* 77(13):1276–82.

Tiemeier, Henning, H. Ruud van Tuijl, Albert Hofman, John Meijer, Amanda J. Kiliaan and Monique M. Breteler. 2002. "Vitamin B_{12}, Folate, and Homocysteine in Depression: the Rotterdam Study." *American Journal of Psychiatry* 159(12):2099–101.

U.S. Department of Agriculture, Agricultural Research Service. 2012. "USDA National Nutrient Database for Standard Reference, Release 25." www.ars.usda.gov/Services/docs.htm?docid=8964

Vogiatzoglou, Anna, David Smith, Eha Nurk, et al. 2013. "Cognitive Function in an Elderly Population: Interaction Between Vitamin B_{12} Status, Depression, and Apolipoprotein E ε4: The Hordaland Homocysteine Study." *Psychosomatic Medicine* 75(1):20–9.

CHAPTER 7

Barragan-Rodriguez, Lazaro, Martha Rodriguez-Moran and Fernando Guerrero-Romero. 2007. "Depressive Symptoms and Hypomagnesemia in Older Diabetic Subjects." *Archives of Medical Research* 38(7):752–6.

Bedford, Jennifer L. and Susan I. Barr. 2011. "Higher Urinary Sodium, a Proxy for Intake, Is Associated with Increased Calcium Excretion and Lower Hip Bone Density in Healthy Young Women with Lower Calcium Intakes." *Nutrients* (3)11:951–61.

Bertone-Johnson, Elizabeth R., Susan E. Hankinson, Adrianne Johnson, Susan R. Bendich, Walter C. Willett and JoAnn E. Manson. 2005. "Calcium and Vitamin D Intake and Risk of Incident Premenstrual Syndrome." *Archives of Internal Medicine* 165(11):1246–52.

Derom, Marie-Laure, Carmen Sayon-Orea, Jose Maria Martinez-Ortega and Miguel Martinez-Gonzalez. 2013. "Magnesium and Depression: A Systematic Review." *Nutritional Neuroscience* 16(5):191–206.

Heaney, Robert P. 2006. "Role of Dietary Sodium in Osteoporosis." *Journal of the American College of Nutrition* 25(3 Suppl):271S–276S.

Hedayati, S. Susan, Abu T. Minhajuddin, Adeel Ijaz, et al. 2012. "Association of Urinary Sodium/Potassium Ratio with Blood Pressure: Sex and Racial Differences." *Clinical Journal of the American Society of Nephrology* 7(2):315–22.

Huang, Jui-Hua, Yi-Fa Lu, Fu-Chou Cheng, Lee Cheng, N.Y. John and Leih-Ching Tsai. 2012. "Correlation of Magnesium Intake with Metabolic Parameters, Depression and Physical Activity in Elderly Type 2 Diabetes Patients: A Cross-Sectional Study." *Nutrition Journal* 11:41.

Joo, Nam-Seok, Bess Dawson-Hughes, Young-Sang Kim, Kyungwon Oh and Kyung-Jin Yeum. 2012. "Impact of Calcium and Vitamin D Insufficiencies on Serum Parathyroid Hormone and Bone Mineral Density: Analysis of the Fourth and Fifth Korea National Health and Nutrition Examination Survey (KNHAENS IV-3, 2009 and V-1, 2010)." *Journal of Bone and Mineral Research* 28(4):764–70.

Kim, Soon-Kyung and Yun-Jung Bae. 2012. "Low Dietary Calcium is Associated with Self-Rated Depression in Middle-Aged Korean Women." *Nutrition Research and Practice* 6(6):527–33.

Laires, Maria Jose and Christina Monteiro. 2008. "Exercise, Magnesium and Immune Function." *Magnesium Research* 21(2):92–6.

Lanham-New, Susan A. 2008. "The Balance of Bone Health: Tipping the Scales in Favor of Potassium-Rich, Bicarbonate-Rich Foods." *The Journal of Nutrition* 138(1):172S–75S.

Li, Xiu-Yang, Xian-Lei Cai and Ping-Da Bian. 2012. "High Salt Intake and Stroke: Meta-Analysis of the Epidemiologic Evidence." *CNS Neuroscience & Therapeutics* 18(8):691–701.

Lukaski, Henry C. and Forrest H. Nielsen. 2002. "Dietary Magnesium Depletion Affects Metabolic Responses during Submaximal Exercise in Postmenopausal Women." *Journal of Nutrition* 132(5):930–5.

Millward, D. Joe. 2012. "Nutrition and Sarcopenia: Evidence for an Interaction." *Proceedings of the Nutrition Society* 71(4):566–75.

Peterlik, Meinrad, Enikoe Kallay and Heide S. Cross. 2013. "Calcium Nutrition and Extracellular Calcium Sensing: Relevance for the Pathogenesis of Osteoporosis, Cancer and Cardiovascular Diseases." *Nutrients* 5(1):302–27.

Seo, Mi Hae, Mee Kyoung Kim and Se Eun Park. 2013. "The Association Between Daily Calcium Intake and Sarcopenia in Older, Non-Obese Korean Adults: the Fourth Korea National Health and Nutrition Examination Survey (KNHANES IV) 2009." *Endocrine Journal* 60(5):679–86.

Torres, Susan J., Caryl A. Nowson and Anthony Worsley. 2008. "Dietary Electrolytes are Related to Mood." *British Journal of Nutrition* 100(5):1038–45.

U.S. Department of Agriculture, Agricultural Research Service. 2012. "Energy Intakes: Percentages of Energy from Protein, Carbohydrate, Fat, and Alcohol, by Gender and Age, What We Eat in America, NHANES 2009–2010." www.ars.usda.gov/ba/bhnrc/fsrg

U.S. Department of Agriculture, Agricultural Research Service. 2012. "USDA National Nutrient Database for Standard Reference, Release 25." www.ars.usda.gov/Services/docs.htm?docid=8964

Yang, Quanhe, Tiebin Liu, Elana Kuklina, et al. 2011. "Sodium and Potassium Intake and Mortality Among US Adults: Prospective Data From the Third National Health and Nutrition Examination Survey." *Archives of Internal Medicine* 71(13):1183–91.

Yary, Teymoor, Sanaz Aazami and Kourosh, Soleimannejad. 2012. "Dietary Intake of Magnesium May Modulate Depression." *Biological Trace Element Research* 151(3):324–9.

Zhu, Kun, Amanda Devine, Richard L. Prince. 2009. "The Effects of High Potassium Consumption On Bone Mineral Density in a Prospective Cohort Study of Elderly Postmenopausal Women." *Osteoporosis International* 20(2):335–40.

CHAPTER 8

Al Mofleh, Ibrahim Abdulkarim. 2010. "Spices, Herbal Xenobiotics and the Stomach: Friends or Foes?" *World Journal of Gastroenterology* 16(22):2710–9.

Al-Safi, Saafan A., Nehad M. Ayoub, Imad Al-Doghim, and Faisal Aboul-Enein. 2011. "Dark Chocolate and Blood Pressure: A Novel Study From Jordan." *Current Drug Delivery* 8(6):595–9.

Boeing, Heiner, Angela Bechthold, Achim Bub, et al. 2012. "Critical Review: Vegetables and Fruit in the Prevention of Chronic Diseases." *European Journal of Nutrition* 51(6):637–63.

Cosgrove, Maeve C., Oscar H. Franco, Stewart P. Granger, Peter G. Murray and Andrew E. Mayes. 2007. "Dietary Nutrient Intakes and Skin-Aging Appearance Among Middle-Aged American Women." *American Journal of Clinical Nutrition* 86(4):1225–31.

Djousse, Luc, Paul Hopkins, Kari North, James Pankow, Donna Arnett and R. Curtis Ellison. 2011. "Chocolate Consumption is Inversely Associated with Prevalent Coronary Heart Disease: the National Heart, Lung, and Blood Institute Family Heart Study." *Clinical Nutrition* 30(2):182–7.

Evans, Julie A. and Elizabeth J. Johnson. 2010. "The Role of Phytonutrients in Skin Health." *Nutrients* 2(8):903–28.

Halvorsen, Bente L., Monica H. Carlsen, Katherine M. Phillips, et al. 2006. "Content of Redox-Active Compounds (ie, antioxidants) in Foods Consumed in the United States." *American Journal of Clinical Nutrition* 84(1):95–13.

Hooper, Lee, Colin Kay, Asmaa Abdelhamid, et al. 2012. "Effects of Chocolate, Cocoa, and Flavan-3-ols on Cardiovascular Health: A Systematic Review and Meta-Analysis of Randomized Trials." *American Journal of Clinical Nutrition* 95(3):740–51.

Kang, Jae H., Alberto Ascherio and Francine Grodstein. 2005. "Fruit and Vegetable Consumption and Cognitive Decline in Aging Women." *Annals of Neurology* 57(5):713–20.

Katz, David L., Kim Doughty and Ather Ali. 2011. "Cocoa and Chocolate in Human Health and Disease." *Antioxidants & Redox Signaling* 15(10):2779–811.

Kemps, Eva and Marika Tiggemann. 2013. "Olfactory Stimulation Curbs Food Cravings." *Addictive Behavior* 38(2):1550–4.

Kemps, Eva, Marika Tiggemann and Sarah Bettany. 2012. "Non-Food Odorants Reduce Chocolate Cravings." *Appetite* 58(3):1087–90.

Lee, Roberta and Michael J. Balick. 2001. "Chocolate: Healing 'Food of the Gods'?" *Alternative Therapies Health Medicine* 7(5):120–2.

Loef, M. and Walach Harold. 2012. "Fruit, Vegetables and Prevention of Cognitive Decline or Dementia: a Systematic Review of Cohort Studies." *Journal of Nutrition, Health & Aging* 16(7):626–30.

Martin, François-Pierre J., Nicholas Antille, Serge Rezzi and Sunil Kochhar. 2012. "Everyday Eating Experiences of Chocolate and Non-Chocolate Snacks Impact Postprandial Anxiety, Energy and Emotional States." *Nutrients* 4(6):554–67.

Palmer, Sharon. 2012. *The Plant-Powered Diet: The Lifelong Eating Plan for Achieving Optimal Health, Beginning Today*. New York: The Experiment.

Panickar, Kiran. 2012. "Beneficial Effects of Herbs, Spices, and Medicinal Plants on the Metabolic Syndrome, Brain, and Cognitive Function." *Central Nervous System Agents in Medicinal Chemistry* 13(1):13–29.

Pase, Matthew P., Andrew B. Scholey, Andrew Pipingas, et al. 2013. "Cocoa Polyphenols Enhance Positive Mood States but Not Cognitive Performance: A Randomized, Placebo-Controlled Trial." *Journal of Psychopharmacology* 27(5):451–8.

Polidori, M. Christina, Domenico Practico, Francesca Mangialasche, et al. 2009. "High Fruit and Vegetable Intake is Positively Correlated With Antioxidant Status and Cognitive Performance in Healthy Subjects." *Journal of Alzheimer's Disease* 17(4):921–7.

Ried, K., T.R. Sullivan, P. Fakler, O.R. Frank and N.P. Stocks. "Effect of cocoa on blood pressure." *Cochrane Database of Systematic Reviews* 2010, Issue 12. Art. No.: CD008893. doi:10.1002/14651858. CD008893.

Sabia, Severine, Archana Singh-Manoux, Gareth Hagger-Johnson, Emmanuelle Cambios, Eric J. Brunner and Mika Kivimaki. 2012. "Influence of Individual and Combined Healthy Behaviours on Successful Aging." *Canadian Medical Association Journal* 184(18):1985–92.

Taubert, Dirk, Renate Roesen and Edgar Schomig. 2007. "Effect of Cocoa and Tea Intake on Blood Pressure: a Meta-Analysis." *Archives of Internal Medicine* 167(7):626–34.

Tokede, O.A., J.M. Gaziano and L. Djousse. 2011. "Effects of Cocoa Products/Dark Chocolate on Serum Lipids: a Meta-analysis." *European Journal of Clinical Nutrition* 65(8):879–86.

U.S. Department of Agriculture, Agricultural Research Service. 2012. "Energy Intakes: Percentages of Energy from Protein, Carbohydrate, Fat, and Alcohol, by Gender and Age, What We Eat in America, NHANES 2009–2010." www.ars.usda.gov/ba/bhnrc/fsrg

Weaver, Connie M., Lee D. Alekel, Wendy E. Ward and Martin J. Ronis. 2012. "Flavonoid Intake and Bone Health." *Journal of Nutrition in Gerontology and Geriatrics* 31(3):239–53.

Whitehead, Ross D., Daniel Re, Dengke Xiao, Gozde Ozakinci and David I. Perrett. 2012. "You Are What You Eat: Within-Subject Increases In Fruit and Vegetable Consumption Confer Beneficial Skin-Color Changes." *PLoS One* 7(3):e32988.

CHAPTER 9

Arab, Lenore, Weiging Liu and David Elashoff. 2009. "Green and Black Tea Consumption and Risk of Stroke: a Meta-Analysis." *Stroke* 40(5):1786–92.

Armstrong, Lawrence, Matthew Ganio, Douglas J. Casa, et al. 2012. "Mild Dehydration Affects Mood in Healthy Young Women." *The Journal of Nutrition* 142(2):382–8.

Bahorun, Theeshan, Amitabye Luximon-Ramma, Vidushi S. Neergheen-Bhujun, et al. 2012. "The Effect of Black Tea on Risk Factors of Cardiovascular Disease in a Normal Population." *Preventive Medicine* 54(1):S98–S102.

Beverage Marketing. "Press Release: Bottled Water Shows Strength Yet Again, New Report From BMC Shows." Accessed June 13, 2013, www.beveragemarketing.com/news-detail.asp?id=260

Bryan, Janet. 2008. "Psychological Effects of Dietary Components of Tea: Caffeine and L-Theanine." *Nutrition Reviews* 66(2):82–90.

Butt, Masood Sadiq and M. Tauseef Sultan. 2011. "Coffee and its Consumption: Benefits and Risks." *Critical Reviews in Food Science Nutrition* 51(4):363–73.

Chen, Honglei. "Hold the Diet Soda? Sweetened Drinks Linked to Depression, Coffee Tied to Lower Risk" (lecture). American Academy of Neurology's 65th Annual Meeting, San Diego, CA, March 16–23, 2013.

Davy, Brenda M., Elizabeth A. Dennis, A. Laura Dengo, Kelly L. Wilson and Kevin P. Davy. 2008. "Water Consumption Reduces Energy Intake at a Breakfast Meal in Obese Older Adults." *Journal of the American Dietetic Association* 108(7):1236–39.

De Koning Gans, J. Margot, Cuno C.S. Uiterwaal, Yvonne T. Van Der Schouw, et al. 2010. "Tea and Coffee Consumption and Cardiovascular Morbidity and Mortality." *Arteriosclerosis, Thrombosis, and Vascular Biology* 30:1665–71.

Dennis, Elizabeth, Ana Laura Dengo, Dana L. Comber, et al. 2010. "Water Consumption Increases Weight Loss During a Hypocaloric Diet Intervention in Middle-Aged and Older Adults." *Obesity* 18(2):300–7.

Elwood, Peter C., Janet E. Pickering, D. Ian Givens and John E. Gallacher. 2010. "The Consumption of Milk and Dairy Foods and the Incidence of Vascular Disease and Diabetes: an Overview of the Evidence." *Lipids* 45(10):925–39.

Ernst, Abel, Susan Hendrix, S. Gene McNeeley, et al. 2007. "Daily Coffee Consumption and Prevalence of Nonmelanoma Skin Cancer in Caucasian Women." *European Journal of Cancer Prevention* 16(5):446–52.

Fletcher, Anne M. 2002. *Sober For Good: New Solutions for Drinking Problems—Advice From Those Who Have Succeeded.* Boston: Houghton Mifflin Harcourt.

Freedman, Neal, Yikyung Park, Christian Abnet, Albert Hollenbeck and Rashmi Sinha. 2012. "Association of Coffee Drinking with Total and Cause-Specific Mortality." *New England Journal of Medicine* 366:1891–1904.

Hegarty, Verona M., Helen M. May and Kay-Tee Khaw. 2000. "Tea Drinking and Bone Mineral Density in Older Women." *American Journal of Clinical Nutrition* 71(4):1003–7.

Heinrich, Ulrike, Caroline E. Moore, Silke De Spirit, Hagen Tronnier and Wilhelm Stahl. 2011. "Green Tea Polyphenols Provide Photoprotection, Increase Microcirculation, and Modulate Skin Properties of Women." *Journal of Nutrition* 141(6):1202–8.

Higdon, Jane V. and Baiz Frei. 2006. "Coffee and Health: a Review of Recent Human Research." *Critical Reviews in Food Science Nutrition* 46(2):101–23.

Hozawa, Atsushi, Shinichi Kuriyama and Naoki Nakaya. 2009. "Green Tea Consumption is Associated with Lower Psychological Distress in a General Population: the Ohsaki Cohort 2006 Study." *American Journal of Clinical Nutrition* 90(5):1390–6.

Kleiner, Susan. 1999. "Water: An Essential But Overlooked Nutrient." *Journal of the American Dietetic Association* 99(2):200–6.

O'Neil, Carol E., Theresa A. Nicklas, Gail C. Rampersaud and Victor L. Fulgoni III. 2012. "100% Orange Juice Consumption is Associated with Better Diet Quality, Improved Nutrient Adequacy, Decreased Risk for Obesity, and Improved Biomarkers of Health in Adults: National Health and Nutrition Examination Survey, 2003–2006." *Nutrition Journal* 11:107.

Patil, Harshal, Carl Lavie and James O'Keefe. 2011. "Cuppa Joe: Friend or Foe? Effects of Chronic Coffee Consumption on Cardiovascular and Brain Health." *Missouri Medicine* 108(6):431–8.

Peters, Ulrike, Charles Poole, Lenore Arba. 2001. "Does Tea Affect Cardiovascular Disease? A Meta-Analysis." *American Journal of Epidemiology* 154(6):495–503.

Song, Fengju, Jiali Han and Abrar A. Qureshi. 2012. "Increased Caffeine Intake is Associated with Reduced Risk of Basal Cell Carcinoma of the Skin." *Cancer Research* 72(13):3282–9.

Steptoe, Andrew, E. Leigh Gibson, Raisa Vounonvirta. 2007. "The Effects of Tea on Psychophysiological Stress Responsivity and Post-Stress Recovery: A Randomised Double-Blind Trial." *Psychopharmacology* 190(1):81–9.

Van Walleghen, Emily L., Jeb S. Orr, Chris L. Gentile, and Brenda M. Davy. 2007. "Pre-meal Water Consumption Reduces Meal Energy Intake in Older But Not Younger Subjects." *Obesity* 15(1):93–9.

Vernarelli, Jacqueline A. and Joshua D. Lambert. 2012. "Tea Consumption is Inversely Associated with Weight Status and Other Markers for Metabolic Syndrome in US Adults." *European Journal of Nutrition* 52(3):1039–48.

Zemel, Michael. 2009. "Proposed Role of Calcium and Dairy Food Components in Weight Management and Metabolic Health." *The Physician and Sports Medicine* 37(2):29–39.

CHAPTER 10

Catenacci, Victoria A., Gary K. Grunwald, Jan P. Ingebrigtsen, et al. 2011. "Physical Activity Patterns Using Accelerometry in the National Weight Control Registry." *Obesity* 19(6):1163–70.

Coon, Jo Thompson, Kate Boddy, Ken Stein, R. Whear, J. Barton and M.H. Depledge. 2011. "Does Participating in Physical Activity in Outdoor Natural Environments Have a Greater Effect on Physical and Mental Wellbeing than Physical Activity Indoors? A Systematic Review." *Environmental Science and Technology* 45(5):1761–72.

Gerber, Markus and Uwe Puhse. 2009. "Review Article: Do Exercise and Fitness Protect Against Stress-Induced Health Complaints? A Review of the Literature." *Scandinavian Journal of Public Health* 37(8):801–19.

Hanlon, Bliss, Michael J. Larson, Bruce W. Bailey and James D. Lecheminant. 2012. "Neural Response to Pictures of Food After Exercise in Normal-Weight and Obese Women." *Medicine & Science in Sports and Exercise* 44(10):1864–70.

Joen, Christie Y., R. Peter Lokken, Frank B. Hu and Rob M. van Dam. 2007. "Physical Activity of Moderate Intensity and Risk of Type 2 Diabetes: A Systematic Review." *Diabetes Care* 30(3):744–52.

Kelley, George A., Kristi S. Kelley and Wendy M. Kohrt. 2013. "Exercise and Bone Mineral Density in Premenopausal Women: A Meta-Analysis of Randomized Controlled Trials." *International Journal of Endocrinology* doi:10.1155/2013/741639.

Kline, Christopher E., Xuemei Sui, Martica H. Hall, et al. 2012. "Dose–Response Effects of Exercise Training on the Subjective Sleep Quality of Postmenopausal Women: Exploratory Analyses of a Randomised Controlled Trial." *British Medical Journal* 2:e001044.

Knauper, Barebel, Rowena Pillay, Julien Lacaille, Amanda McCollam and Evan Kelso. 2011. "Replacing Craving Imagery With Alternative Pleasant Imagery Reduces Craving Intensity." *Appetite* 57(1):173–8.

Mengmeng, Du, Jennifer Prescott, Peter Kraft, et al. 2012. "Physical Activity, Sedentary Behavior, and Leukocyte Telomere Length in Women." *American Journal of Epidemiology* 175(5):414–22.

National Center for Health Statistics. 2011. *Health, United States, 2010: With Special Feature on Death and Dying*. Hyattsville, MD.

Oh, Hwajung and Adrian Taylor. 2012. "Brisk Walking Reduces Ad Libitum Snacking in Regular Chocolate Eaters During a Workplace Simulation." *Appetite* 58(1):387–92.

O'Keefe, James and Carl Lavie. 2012. "Run For Your Life ... at a Comfortable Speed and Not Too Far." *British Medical Journal* doi:10.1136/heartjnl-2012–302886.

Palasuwan, Attakorn, Daroonwan Suksom, Irene Margaritis, Suphan Soogarun and Anne-Sophie Rousseau. 2011. "Effects of Tai Chi Training on Antioxidant Capacity in Pre- and Postmenopausal Women." *Journal of Aging Research* 2011:234696.

Passos, Giselle Soares, Dalva Lucia Rollemberg Poyares, Marcos Goncalves Santana, Sergio Tufik and Marco Tulio de Mello. 2012. "Is Exercise an Alternative Treatment for Chronic Insomnia?" *Clinics* 67(6):653–60.

Pavey, Toby G., Geeske Peeters and Wendy J. Brown. 2012. "Sitting-Time and 9-Year All-Cause Mortality in Older Women." *British Journal of Sports and Medicine* doi:10.1136/bjsports-2012–0916761.

Plante, Thomas G., Carissa Gustafson, Carrie Brecht, Jenny Imberi, Jacqueline Sanchez. 2011. "Exercising with an iPod, Friend, or Neither: Which is Better for Psychological Benefits?" *American Journal of Health Behavior* 35(2):199–208.

Puetz, Timothy W., Patrick J. O'Connor and Rod K. Dishman. 2008. "A Randomized Controlled Trial of the Effect of Aerobic Exercise Training on Feelings of Energy and Fatigue in Sedentary Young Adults with Persistent Fatigue." *Psychotherapy and Psychosomatics* 77(3):167–74.

Puterman, Eli, Jue Lin, Elizabeth Blackburn, Aoife O'Donovan, Nancy Adler and Elissa Epel. 2010. "The Power of Exercise: Buffering the Effect of Chronic Stress on Telomere Length." *PLoS One* 5(5):e10837.

Rebholz, Casey M., Dongfeng Gu, Jing Chen, et al. 2012. "Physical Activity Reduces Salt Sensitivity of Blood Pressure: The Genetic Epidemiology Network of Salt Sensitivity Study." *American Journal of Epidemiology* 1:176.

Ross, Alyson and Sue Thomas. 2010. "The Health Benefits of Yoga and Exercise: a Review of Comparison Studies." *The Journal of Alternative and Complementary Medicine* 16(1):3–12.

Sattelmair, Jacob, Jeremy Pertman, Eric L. Ding, Harold W. Kohl III, William Haskell and I-Min Lee. 2011. "Dose Response Between Physical Activity and Risk of Coronary Heart Disease: A Meta-Analysis." *Circulation* 124(7):789–95.

Schnohr, P. 2012. "Regular Jogging Shows Dramatic Increase in Life Expectancy" (lecture). MP3 from European Society of Cardiology. Recorded at EuroPRevent in Dublin, Ireland. May 5th, 2012.

Uchida, Sunao, Kohei Shioda, Yuko Morita, Chie Kubota, Masashi Ganeko and Noriko Takeda. 2012. "Exercise Effects on Sleep Physiology." *Frontiers in Neurology* 3:48.

U.S. Department of Health & Human Services. "2008 Physical Activity Guidelines for Americans." Accessed February 15, 2013. www.health.gov/paguidelines

Van der Ploeg, Hidde P., Tien Chey, Rosemmary J. Korda, Emily Banks and Adrian Bauman. 2012. "Sitting Time and All-Cause Mortality Risk in 222 497 Australian Adults." *Archives of Internal Medicine* 172(6):494–500.

Woods, Nancy Fugate, Ellen Sullivan Mitchell and Kathy Smith-Di Julio. 2010. "Sexual Desire During the Menopausal Transition and Early Postmenopause: Observations from the Seattle Midlife Women's Health Study." *Journal of Women's Health* 19(2):209–18.

Yang, Pei Yu, Ka-Hou Ho, His-Chung Chen and Meng-Yueh Chien. 2012. "Exercise Training Improves Sleep Quality in Middle-Aged and Older Adults With Sleep Problems: a Systematic Review." *Journal of Physiotherapy* 58(3):157–63.

CHAPTER 11

Afaghi, Ahmad, Helen O'Connor and Chin Moi Chow. 2007. "High-Glycemic-Index Carbohydrate Meals Shorten Sleep Onset." *American Journal of Clinical Nutrition* 85(2):426–30.

American Psychological Association. "Stress in America Survey." Accessed March 30, 2013. www.apa.org/news/press/releases/stress/index.aspx

Arnedt, J. Todd, Damaris J. Rohsenow and Alissa B. Almeida. 2011. "Sleep Following Alcohol Intoxication in Healthy, Young Adults: Effects of Sex and Family History of Alcoholism." *Alcoholism Clinical and Experimental Research* 35(5):870–8.

Buckley, Theresa and Alan F. Schatzberg. 2005. "On the Interactions of the Hypothalamic-Pituitary-Adrenal (HPA) Axis and Sleep: Normal HPA Axis Activity and Circadian Rhythm, Exemplary Sleep Disorders." *The Journal of Clinical Endocrinology & Metabolism* 90(5):3106–114.

Cappuccio, Francesco, Daniel Cooper, Lanfranco D'Elia, Pasquale Strazzullo and Michelle Miller. 2011. "Sleep Duration Predicts Cardiovascular Outcomes: A Systematic Review and Meta-Analysis of Prospective Studies." *European Heart Journal* 32:1484–92.

Chaput, Jean-Philippe, Jean-Pierre Despres, Claude Bouchard and Angelo Tremblay. 2008. "The Association Between Sleep Duration and Weight Gain in Adults: A 6-Year Prospective Study from the Quebec Family Study." *Sleep* 31(4):517–23.

Howatson, Glyn, Phillip G. Bell, Jamie Tallent, Benita Middleton, Malachy P. McHugh and Jason Ellis. 2012. "Effect of Tart Cherry Juice (Prunus cerasus) on Melatonin Levels and Enhanced Sleep Quality." *European Journal of Nutrition* 51(8):909–16.

Neckelmann, Dag, Arnstein Mykletun and Alv A. Dahl. 2007. "Chronic Insomnia as a Risk Factor for Developing Anxiety and Depression." *Sleep* 30(7)873–80.

Patel, Sanjay R., Atul Malhotra, David P. White, Daniel J. Gottlieb and Frank B. Hu. 2006. "Association Between Reduced Sleep and Weight Gain in Women." *American Journal of Epidemiology* 164(10):947–54.

Peuhkuri, Katri, Nora Sihvola and Riitta Korpela. 2012. "Dietary factors and fluctuating levels of melatonin." *Food and Nutrition Research* 56. doi:10.3402/fnr.v56i0.17252.

Somer, Elizabeth. 2009. *Eat Your Way to Happiness*. Toronto:Harlequin.

ACKNOWLEDGMENTS

I have many people to thank for helping to make *Younger Next Week* a reality. Thank you to my friend Keri Gans for introducing me to the smart and savvy Celeste Fine, who supported me and enriched my book idea from the get-go. To the wonderful Frances Sharpe, who partnered with me to craft a terrific book proposal. To my incredible team at Harlequin Nonfiction for putting together a beautiful book: Sarah Pelz, for her enthusiasm for my book from the start and for her incredible support during the book-writing process; Rosemary Silva for copyediting so brilliantly; Shara Alexander and Lathea Williams for the incredible publicity support; and Merjane Schouri, Diane Mosher and Fiona Cunningham for their marketing mojo. Special thanks also go to my dear friend Elaine Friedman, for her amazing editing (and cheerleading) skills, and to Susan Male, for being the best technical editor a girl can ask for. And to Robyn Webb, MS, for her incredible Vital Recipes.

A big thank-you to Jillian Meshnick for her invaluable help running my office and seeing the book come to fruition, and for always having a smile on her face. Special thanks also go to all the terrific dietetic interns and students with whom I've had the pleasure to work over the past two years, including Stacy Abbatiello, Briana Adler, Erika Breitfeller, Lauren Cagliostro, Gina Gabbamonte, Gary Kwo, Carly Levine, Kristy Logan, Kristen Mannix, Alyce Manzo, Stefani Pappas, Kayla Reinstein and Aimee Zipkin.

Thanks also go out to my stellar branding team, Mitchell Stewart, Paul Heyman, Enersy Mendez, Lauren Choinski, Jordan Baker Caldwell, Renee Arochas and Many Wherthenschlag for their talent, enthusiasm, support and encouragement.

A special thank-you to the scores of friends, neighbors, clients and consumers who shared their stories with me, took a survey, participated in a test panel or otherwise provided feedback to help make *Younger Next Week* better. And a special thank-you to Tracy Minucci, for her friendship and for reading my manuscript, and to two of my BFFs—Cheryl Harris and Allison Gelfman—for cheering me on through the book-writing process. And to my other BFF, Zari Ginsburg, and her children, Sydney, Alana and Evan, thanks for all the brown rice and starchy carb memories. And to Maria Arevalo for enabling me to work full-time while raising my two children. Te amo, Li Li!

I'd like to also thank all of the following colleagues and friends who took time to lend their expertise to make *Younger Next Week* even better: Kelly Allison, PhD; Karen Ansel, MS, RD, CDN; Lawrence E. Armstrong, PhD; Patricia Bannan, MS, RD; Joy Bauer, MS, RD; Rachel Begun, MS, RD, CDN; Janice Newell Bissex, MS, RD; Janet Brill, RD, PhD; Jeffrey Blumberg, PhD; Laura Cipullo, RD, CDN; Karen Collins, MS, RDN, CDN; Aimee Crant-Oksa, MS, RD; Michelle Dudash, RD; Ann Fletcher, MS, RD, LD; Cheryl Forberg, RD; Kate Geagan, MS, RD; Andrea Giancoli, MPH, RD; Tara Gidus, MS, RD; Michael Grandner, PhD; David Grotto, RD, LDN; Cheryl Harris, MPH, RD; Marla Heller, MS, RD; Samantha Heller, RD; Janet Helm, MS, RD; Cindy Heroux, RD; James O. Hill,

PhD; David L. Katz, MD; Kristin McGee; Julie Meyer, RD; Lisa Morse, PhD; Elana Tapper Natker, MS, RD; Jackie Newgent, RD, CDN; Sharon Palmer, MS, RD; Silsbee Philo; Yvette Rivera; Barbara Rolls, PhD; Kate Scarlata, RD; Lauren Slayton, MS, RD; Meredith Sobel, MS, RD, CDN; Elizabeth Somer, MA, RD; Bethany Thayer, MS, RD; Evelyn Tribole, MS, RD; Joe Vinson, PhD; Liz Weiss, MS, RD; Delia Willsey; Vonda Wright, MD; Judith J. Wurtman, PhD; and Lisa Young, PhD, RD.

Finally, I'd like to thank my beautiful family for making my life that much sweeter. They are my everything.

INDEX

ABOUT THE AUTHOR

Nationally recognized registered dietitian nutritionist Elisa Zied has shared her food, nutrition and fitness expertise and her real-world approach to behavior and lifestyle change with consumers for nearly two decades. A past national media spokesperson for the Academy of Nutrition and Dietetics, a title she held for six years, Elisa has garnered millions of media impressions and has been featured on dozens of television programs, including *The Today Show* and *Good Morning America*. She was also a regular on-air contributor to *The Early Show* for more than three years. She is frequently quoted in magazines and newspapers, including *People, Reader's Digest, Shape, Ladies' Home Journal, Parenting, Fitness, Self, Redbook, Prevention, O, More, Women's Health,* the *Wall Street Journal,* the *New York Times,* the *Chicago Tribune,* the *Washington Post* and *USA Today,* and on websites, including WebMD.com and Forbes.com.

Elisa is a regular contributor to *U.S. News & World Report's Eat + Run* blog, NBCNews. com, Caloriecount.com and Galtime.com. She is also on the advisory board of *Parents* magazine, pens a Q&A for Parents.com and writes the popular twice weekly blog on Parents.com called *The Scoop on Food*. Her articles have also appeared in *Parents, Redbook, Seventeen, Woman's Day, Weight Watchers* and *Food & Nutrition* magazines.

Elisa is the author of the award-winning book *Nutrition at Your Fingertips* (Alpha, 2009) and coauthor, with Ruth Winter, MS, of *Feed Your Family Right!* (Wiley, 2007) and *So What Can I Eat?!* (Wiley, 2006). Elisa has also been a keynote or featured speaker at several events for both professionals and consumers, and she has worked as a spokesperson for products that align with her message. She is also the recipient of the 2007 New York State Dietetic Association Media Excellence Award.

Elisa is a proud member of the Academy of Nutrition and Dietetics and several of its practice groups, including Women's Health, Weight Management, Dietitians in Business and Communications, Nutrition Entrepreneurs and Pediatrics. She is also on the advisory board of Live Light Live Right, an obesity prevention program that serves low-income children and is based in Brooklyn, New York.

Elisa earned a bachelor of arts in psychology from the University of Pennsylvania and a master of science in clinical nutrition from New York University. She has maintained her certification as a personal trainer by the American Council on Exercise since 1994.

In 2010 Elisa founded Zied Health Communications, LLC, a food and nutrition communications firm. She lives and works in New York City with her husband of more than twenty years and their two sons, aged fifteen and twelve. Elisa maintains an active and healthy lifestyle by power walking, hula hooping, dancing, weight training and running around with her boys. She relies on her Jawbone UP bracelet to count her steps and loves chocolate, Brussels sprouts and pink grapefruits.

Visit www.elisazied.com to learn more about Elisa, to join her mailing list and to have access to helpful Stressipes and delicious recipes, and other tips and tools to help you eat and live better.